Understanding Yourself and Others

Bob Thomson is an experienced coach and management development professional. He currently works as a Professor of Practice at Warwick Business School. He established the University of Warwick's Certificate and Diploma in Coaching, and set up the University's MA in Coaching through action learning. He was formerly Leadership Development Manager at National Grid Transco.

Bob has written a number of other books on coaching and on learning and development:

- *Growing People: Learning and developing from day to day experience*
- *Don't Just Do Something, Sit There: An introduction to non-directive coaching*
- *The Coaching Dance: A tale of coaching and management*
- *Non-directive Coaching: Attitudes, approaches and applications*
- *First Steps in Coaching.*

Don't Just Do Something, Sit There was published in Chinese under the title *Modern Midwifery: The art of coaching*, which reflects the notion of Socratic questioning.

He may be contacted by email at <bob.thomson@wbs.ac.uk>

Overcoming Common Problems Series

Selected titles

A full list of titles is available from Sheldon Press,
36 Causton Street, London SW1P 4ST and on our website at
www.sheldonpress.co.uk

101 Questions to Ask Your Doctor
Dr Tom Smith

Asperger Syndrome in Adults
Dr Ruth Searle

The Assertiveness Handbook
Mary Hartley

Assertiveness: Step by step
Dr Windy Dryden and Daniel Constantinou

Backache: What you need to know
Dr David Delvin

Birth Over 35
Sheila Kitzinger

Body Language: What you need to know
David Cohen

Breast Cancer: Your treatment choices
Dr Terry Priestman

Bulimia, Binge-eating and their Treatment
Professor J. Hubert Lacey, Dr Bryony Bamford
and Amy Brown

The Cancer Survivor's Handbook
Dr Terry Priestman

The Chronic Pain Diet Book
Neville Shone

Cider Vinegar
Margaret Hills

Coeliac Disease: What you need to know
Alex Gazzola

**Coping Successfully with Chronic Illness:
Your healing plan**
Neville Shone

Coping Successfully with Pain
Neville Shone

Coping Successfully with Prostate Cancer
Dr Tom Smith

Coping Successfully with Shyness
Margaret Oakes, Professor Robert Bor
Dr Carina Eriksen

Coping Successfully with Ulcerative Colitis
Peter Cartwright

Coping Successfully with Varicose Veins
Christine Craggs-Hinton

Coping Successfully with Your Hiatus Hernia
Dr Tom Smith

Coping When Your Child Has Cerebral Palsy
Jill Eckersley

Coping with Anaemia
Dr Tom Smith

Coping with Asthma in Adults
Mark Greener

**Coping with Birth Trauma and Postnatal
Depression**
Lucy Jolin

Coping with Bronchitis and Emphysema
Dr Tom Smith

Coping with Candida
Shirley Trickett

Coping with Chemotherapy
Dr Terry Priestman

Coping with Chronic Fatigue
Trudie Chalder

Coping with Coeliac Disease
Karen Brody

Coping with Diverticulitis
Peter Cartwright

Coping with Drug Problems in the Family
Lucy Jolin

Coping with Dyspraxia
Jill Eckersley

Coping with Early-onset Dementia
Jill Eckersley

Coping with Eating Disorders and Body Image
Christine Craggs-Hinton

Coping with Epilepsy
Dr Pamela Crawford and Fiona Marshall

Coping with Gout
Christine Craggs-Hinton

Coping with Guilt
Dr Windy Dryden

Coping with Headaches and Migraine
Alison Frith

Coping with Heartburn and Reflux
Dr Tom Smith

Coping with Life after Stroke
Dr Mareeni Raymond

**Coping with Life's Challenges: Moving on
from adversity**
Dr Windy Dryden

Overcoming Common Problems Series

Overcoming Common Problems Series

Understanding Yourself
and Others

Practical ideas from the world of coaching

BOB THOMSON

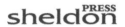
sheldon PRESS

First published in Great Britain in 2014

Sheldon Press
36 Causton Street
London SW1P 4ST
www.sheldonpress.co.uk

The author and publisher have made every effort to ensure that the external
website and email addresses included in this book are correct and up to date at the
time of going to press. The author and publisher are not responsible for the content,
quality or continuing accessibility of the sites.

British Library Cataloguing-in-Publication Data
A catalogue record for this book is available from the British Library

ISBN 978–1–84709–311–0
eBook ISBN 978–1–84709–312–7

Typeset by Caroline Waldron, Wirral, Cheshire
First printed in Great Britain by Ashford Colour Press
Subsequently digitally reprinted in Great Britain

eBook by Fakenham Photosetting Ltd, Fakenham, Norfolk

Produced on paper from sustainable forests

To Alex, Liz and Georgia

Contents

Illustrations

Preface

In writing this book I want to share with you many of the ideas and models that I introduce regularly into coaching conversations to offer people a useful perspective on their situation. My hope is that seeing things afresh will enable them to respond more effectively to address the challenges they're facing or to achieve the goals that they seek.

This reflects a key principle in coaching which can be summarized in this equation:

$$\text{Awareness} + \text{Responsibility} = \text{Performance}$$

The premise behind the equation is that people who are aware of what they need to do and how to do it, and who also take responsibility for acting appropriately, will perform well. What performance means depends on their situation – it might be hitting a tennis ball, playing the flute, decorating a house or managing a team.

Likewise, I hope that you too will find some of the models a helpful way to think about and then address some of the challenging issues that you face. The chapters include exercises inviting you to try out some of the ideas in your day-to-day life. The experience of doing this – and then reflecting upon and making sense of what happens – can help you to translate the ideas into new and useful behaviours and habits. I imagine that different readers will find different ideas useful to them, and I encourage you to focus on those that will help you personally. It may be helpful to have a notebook handy.

The opening chapter sets out the basic ideas in the primarily non-directive approach to coaching that I use with my clients. It goes on to explore the notion that day-to-day experience – coupled with reflection to make sense of that experience – is the key to developing yourself and helping others to learn new skills and abilities. Throughout the book I'll encourage you to try out the ideas and models offered and to learn by reflecting upon how you get on.

The second chapter looks at emotional intelligence. The key aspects of emotional intelligence – understanding and managing yourself, and understanding and relating effectively to others – are themes which will reappear throughout the book. In a sense, this chapter serves as an overture for the rest of this book on understanding yourself and other people.

Chapter 3 is based on the widely used personality questionnaire, the Myers-Briggs Type Indicator®. Exploring the four dimensions of the MBTI® offers rich ideas for understanding yourself, for appreciating how other people operate, and hence for improving how you handle your interactions with others.

In Chapter 4 we consider a number of ideas from Transactional Analysis (TA) that can help you to understand yourself and your relationships with other people. It describes the key notion in TA – Parent, Adult and Child ego states – and goes on to explore other ideas that flow from this.

Relationships are built on conversations. Chapter 5 explores the four key skills needed to engage in constructive conversations – listening, playing back, questioning and voicing. We also look at how to handle difficult conversations.

Chapter 6 looks at two topics – behaving assertively and handling conflict – in which the ability to be aware of and to manage what is going on within yourself is deeply connected to your ability to interact successfully with others. Difficulties in behaving assertively or the inability to address conflict constructively are common themes that arise in coaching conversations.

In Chapter 7 we consider different styles and approaches that you might use to influence other people effectively. As with other aspects of interpersonal behaviour, it helps to have a range of styles rather than a single approach so that you have flexibility and choice in how you behave.

Chapter 8 on time management invites you to focus on yourself and consider what's most important to you in your work and your life. The key to managing your time is to know your priorities and to spend your time in ways which reflect those priorities. It is as simple – and as difficult – as that!

In Chapter 9 we look at situations where you want to achieve things through the efforts of other people. We consider the notion of balancing concern for completing the task and looking after the people who are doing it, and then extend this to include the importance of managing a team collectively.

In the first part of Chapter 10 we look at some ideas that may help you to prepare for a meeting, conduct the meeting well and follow up effectively after the meeting. We then expand these ideas on what you can do before, during and after a meeting when you are the person chairing it.

Change is a common aspect of life today, and the final chapter looks at coping with and managing change. We describe a number of models that help to make sense of change, inviting you to reflect upon how you cope with changes that affect your life. We go on to consider a number of ideas that may help you if you are the person introducing a change that may affect others.

Thank you to everyone at Sheldon Press, especially Fiona Marshall, Liz Jones and Rima Devereaux, for their encouragement and practical help in the production of the book.

Finally, thanks to my wife, Val, and our children, David, Eleanor, Dominic and Olivia, for their love and support.

1

Coaching and learning from experience

Introduction

In my role I coach academics, administrators and commercial managers who work at the University of Warwick. One of the things which I regularly do in my coaching sessions is to offer people a model or framework to help them make sense of things. In this book I'd like to share various concepts that I use in these coaching conversations in the hope that some of them will be of real, practical benefit to you. Different readers will find different ideas useful to them, and I encourage you to focus on those that you think will be of value to you personally.

In this opening chapter I'll set out some of the basic ideas that underpin the primarily non-directive approach to coaching that I use. We then go on to explore the idea that learning to do something you couldn't do before requires first-hand experience coupled with reflection to make sense of your experience. If you want to translate some of the ideas in the book into new behaviours and habits you will need to try things out in practice and then reflect upon what happens.

What is coaching?

I'd like to begin by clarifying what I mean by coaching. When most people think of a coach they have in mind a sports coach, such as a football manager or a golf professional. I myself take tennis lessons, and my tennis coach has clear views on what good tennis strokes look like, how best to grip the racquet and where to position yourself on the court. And I am happy to listen to his instructions and advice, trying to incorporate these into my game. You might characterize this type of coaching as directive.

There are other approaches to coaching, however. In my own practice I work mainly non-directively. My role is to listen to people and ask questions that help them to clarify what they want to achieve and to consider how they will do this. When coaching, I only occasionally make suggestions and rarely give advice.

There isn't an agreed definition or view of what coaching is. Here is the definition that I use as the basis of my own practice as a coach.

Coaching is a relationship of rapport and trust in which the coach uses their ability to listen, to ask questions and to play back what the client has communicated in order to help the client to clarify what matters to them and to work out what to do to achieve their aspirations.

The definition emphasizes my view that the role of the coach is to help you to articulate your goals and how you will set about achieving them. Non-directive coaching is about facilitating, not instructing, advising or guiding.

The definition also describes the three key conversational skills used in coaching:

- listening to understand the individual and his or her world;
- asking mainly open questions that help the person think;
- playing back what the individual has said or perhaps communicated non-verbally.

In sharing some ideas with you in this book, I won't be able to listen to you or to play back what you're thinking. I will, however, ask you questions throughout to encourage you to explore what these ideas might mean for you.

Awareness and responsibility

As noted in the Preface, another way of looking at non-directive coaching is summarized in this equation:

$$\text{Awareness} + \text{Responsibility} = \text{Performance}$$

The equation is intended to convey the notion that when I'm coaching I'm trying to do two things – to help people become more aware of what they need to do and how to do it, and to encourage them to take responsibility for action. The fundamental premise is that people who are aware of what to do and who take responsibility will perform effectively – whatever performance means in their context. It might be carrying out a home improvement project, setting up a community initiative, playing tennis or finishing a course of study.

Note too that awareness without responsibility is just whingeing. In other words, someone who is aware of what he or she needs to do to address an important issue but who takes no responsibility for acting is simply whingeing.

When I introduce a model or framework in a coaching conversation, my intention is to offer people a fresh way of thinking about their circumstances – to raise their awareness. We can then go on to explore what they might do in response to their changed awareness. I sometimes find it helpful to recast the word 'responsibility' as 'response-ability'.

In the chapters which follow I will explain many of the concepts that I share regularly with my coaching clients. I hope you find that some of these enable you to view your situation differently and so raise your awareness. It is then up to you how you respond in the light of this awareness, and I will pose some questions inviting you to consider your response.

The GROW model

There is one other idea from coaching that I'd like to introduce in this opening chapter. The GROW model is a very practical and widely used framework to structure a conversation that enables another person to think through his or her situation and come up with a plan of action. The GROW model can be summarized as:

Goal	What are you trying to achieve?
Reality	What is currently going on?
Options	What could you do?
Will	What will you do?

I introduce the model here because you can use it to coach yourself by working systematically through the four areas to explore an issue and come up with an action plan. Exercise 1.1 offers a number of questions that you might work through to think in a structured way about a challenge or concern that's facing you. As you read through the book and become aware of issues that you'd like to address, you may like to work through the GROW model to identify actions you wish to take in response.

If you use the GROW framework to organize your thinking, you need to use it flexibly. With some issues you may spend a lot of time clarifying the goal, and indeed sometimes once a problem is stated clearly the solution becomes obvious. With other issues the goal may be clear but the current reality complex and worthy of considerable exploration. Or you may find that there are no practical options to achieve your goal and you need to track back to modify or perhaps abandon the goal.

Exercise 1.1 Questions to expand the GROW model

Goal:
1 What are you trying to achieve?
2 Imagine that you have successfully addressed your issue. What does success look like?
3 And what does success feel like?
4 In regard to this issue, what do you really, really want?

Reality:
1 What is happening that makes this an issue for you?
2 Who is involved?
3 What assumptions are you making?
4 What – if anything – have you already done to address the situation?
5 And what has been the effect of what you have done so far?

Options:
1 What options do you have?
2 What else might you do?
3 If you had absolutely no constraints – of time or money or power or health – what would you do?
4 If you had a really wise friend, what would he or she do in your shoes?

Will:

1 Your answers to the last four questions have generated a set of options. Which options will you actually pursue?
2 For each chosen option, what specifically will you do?
3 What help or support do you need?
4 What deadlines will you set for yourself?
5 What is the first step that you will take?

Learning from experience

One of the benefits that people often gain from coaching – and which you may get from reading this book – is that they learn things. For example, they may learn a new skill, change their way of thinking, develop confidence or break an unhelpful habit.

There are times when an insight that you have in a coaching session is enough to enable you to change your behaviour. Change does sometimes happen quickly. But often change only occurs if you work hard outside the coaching sessions.

I strongly believe that deep and sustained learning – that is, becoming able to do something you couldn't do before – only comes through experience. Experience on its own isn't enough, however. You need to reflect on and make sense of your experience to create knowledge, and this knowledge deepens when you apply it in new situations. As shown in Figure 1.1, you can view this as a learning cycle.

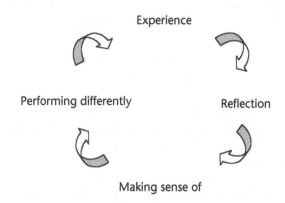

Experience

Performing differently

Reflection

Making sense of

Figure 1.1 The experiential learning cycle

Learning from this book

As you read the various chapters that follow, I hope you find that you'd like to weave some of the models and frameworks into your own way of thinking and behaving. Focusing on the ideas that interest you most, you might like to consider how you can spend time at each of the four points of the learning cycle. The chapters which follow contain exercises inviting you to:

- identify situations where you were either pleased or dissatisfied with how you behaved;
- reflect upon your experiences, or observe how other people do things well;
- consider how an idea can help you to make sense of things;
- try out a new behaviour or experiment with a different approach.

By translating some of these ideas into practice and reflecting upon what then happens, you will hopefully move around the learning cycle and develop new ways of thinking effectively and behaving successfully. If you only read through the ideas explored below, you may find things that interest you but you're unlikely to develop your capability.

Feedback

If you do decide to try out some new ways of thinking and behaving, you might also wish to ask those around you for feedback on how you did. Honest, accurate, specific feedback will raise your awareness of what you're doing well and less well.

Many people aren't very good at giving feedback. Some simply don't notice what you do. Others may notice in general terms but can't articulate what they've observed in useful detail. Some people find it difficult to say anything which might be viewed as critical or negative. And others are all too ready to point out what you've done wrong.

Imagine that you've cooked a meal for some friends and tried out a new recipe. You'd like to know how to improve this dish for next time. You receive these pieces of feedback:

- That was great.
- I didn't enjoy it.
- There was too much garlic and this dominated the taste.

The first two comments may make you feel pleased or disappointed, and are of some interest. However, the third comment is the most useful because it's specific, it describes the effect, and it indicates what you might do differently.

Finding a suitable person to give you useful feedback may not always be feasible. However, as well as asking for feedback, you can also generate your own feedback on how well you've done. Assessing your own performance honestly and realistically will help you to become more aware and prompt you to consider how to respond more effectively next time.

As an illustration, imagine that after reading some of the ideas in later chapters you decide to behave more assertively in certain social situations. You might later reflect on what happened when you tried this by considering questions such as:

- What did I do well in that situation?
- What did I do less well?
- On a scale of 1 to 10, how do I rate my performance?
- What will I do differently next time?
- What have I learnt?

As you experiment with some ideas, I encourage you not to be overly critical of yourself. Rather, keep in mind that you are trying to learn new ways of thinking and behaving, and this may take time. I wish you well!

Exercise 1.2 Reflecting on this chapter

Here are some questions inviting you to consider how you might act at each of the four points of the learning cycle in response to reading this chapter. We begin at the 'Making sense of' position and move round.

- What ideas in this chapter particularly interest you?
- What will you do to try out some of these ideas?

- As you apply these ideas, simply rate your performance on a scale from 1 (very poor) to 10 (excellent).
- After you have tried out an idea, take some time to make a few notes on what went well and what went less well.

2

Emotional intelligence

Introduction

The term 'emotional intelligence' (EI) was popularized in the 1990s by Daniel Goleman, but the idea goes back for centuries. Indeed, Goleman begins his book *Emotional Intelligence* with a quote from the ancient Greek philosopher Aristotle which captures the essence of EI:

> Anyone can become angry – that is easy. But to be angry with the right person, to the right degree, at the right time, for the right purpose, and in the right way – that is not easy.

One of the things which the term 'emotional intelligence' itself did was to legitimize – to some extent, anyway – discussion of feelings in organizations where the main focus was on completing tasks and where discussions were assumed to be based on logic and rational argument.

The key aspects of emotional intelligence – understanding and managing yourself, and understanding and relating effectively to others – are themes which will reappear throughout the book. In a sense, this chapter serves as an overture for the chapters which follow.

A framework for emotional intelligence

I think that the simple framework shown in Figure 2.1 overleaf is a very good way of describing the essence of emotional intelligence. It is based on the notions of awareness and responsibility that we looked at in the opening chapter.

Others	Empathy	Relationship management
Self	Self-awareness	Self-management
	Awareness	Responsibility

Figure 2.1 A framework for emotional intelligence

Self-awareness

The starting point in emotional intelligence – as it is with so many things – is self-awareness. Simply noticing what emotions you are feeling can be very useful.

One thing which helps is to be able to put a name to the emotion that you're feeling – 'I'm sad', 'I feel angry', 'I'm over the moon', and so on. It is very useful to have a vocabulary to name emotions. There are families of emotions – for instance, 'sad, mad, bad and glad' is a simple way of expressing some of the main families of emotions. And then within each family there are different intensities of emotion – for example, 'pleased', 'content', 'happy' and 'delighted' are different intensities within the 'glad' family.

I sometimes imagine a palette of emotions, somewhat similar to the range of colours you are offered when you create a Word or PowerPoint document on your computer. You might consider, for instance, that the red colours represent anger. These can range from a pale pink – mildly irritated – to a deep maroon – incandescent with rage.

One way of naming emotions is simply to find one word which completes the sentence 'I feel . . .' Often, when people begin a sentence 'I feel . . .' they go on to tell you what they think, not what they feel. A useful check is to see whether you can insert the word 'that' after 'I feel' without altering the meaning. If you can, then almost certainly you're dealing with a thought, not a feeling. Compare:

- 'I feel [that] we may miss the train' (a thought).
- 'I feel anxious' (a feeling).

Here is an excerpt from an Ian McEwan novel, *The Innocent*, which describes vividly a character developing self-awareness as he recognizes and names the emotions he is feeling.

Leonard had never in his life spoken about himself and his feelings in such a way. Nor had he even thought in this manner. Quite simply, he had never acknowledged in himself a serious emotion. He had never gone much further than saying he quite liked last night's film, or hated the taste of lukewarm milk. In fact, until now, it was as though he had never really had any serious feelings. Only now, as he came to name them – shame, desperation, love – could he really claim them for his own and experience them. His love for the woman standing by his door was brought into relief by the word, and sharpened the shame he felt for assaulting her. As he gave it a name, the unhappiness of the past three weeks was clarified. He was enlarged, unburdened. Now that he could name the fog he had been moving through, he was at last visible to himself.

As Leonard is able to put a name to his feelings, he becomes 'visible to himself'. In other words, he develops his self-awareness.

Empathy

The other aspect of awareness is awareness of how the other person is feeling, which is often described as empathy. To understand other people empathically is to stand in their shoes, seeing the world from their perspective, appreciating their hopes and aspirations, their concerns and fears.

A vital skill in empathy is the ability to listen attentively, seeking to understand other people. Sometimes they will tell you how they feel, but often they may communicate this non-verbally through their tone of voice, the colour of their cheeks, their gestures or their movements. When you listen to understand another person, you need to look out for what's not being said as well as the words that are spoken. Picking up on emotions that are revealed non-verbally is inevitably more provisional or tentative than picking up on the words that someone says. Having a rich vocabulary that enables you to describe the other person's emotion or emotions accurately is again very useful.

Note that empathy is not the same as sympathy. When you sympathize with someone, you are imagining how you would feel if you were in the same position. When you empathize, you seek to understand how people feel in their situation. As an illustration, let's assume that someone tells you she's just been made redundant. If you were in that position, you might feel very anxious about how you were going to manage on a greatly reduced income. Asking her how she feels might reveal that she is glad to be free of a job she didn't enjoy and is looking forward to making a fresh start in a new career.

Exercise 2.1 Acceptable and unacceptable emotions

I don't actually agree with Aristotle's view that everyone finds it easy to become angry. I think some people find it very, very difficult to become angry, or perhaps to acknowledge to themself that they are indeed angry. Moreover, there are some emotions you may find it easy to accept in other people and some you find it hard to tolerate.

- Which emotions do you freely allow yourself to feel?
- Which emotions do you find it difficult to acknowledge in yourself?
- Which emotions do you readily accept in others?
- Which emotions do you find it difficult to accept in others? How do you respond when you notice these emotions?

Self-management

We move now from awareness – of yourself and others – to responsibility. It isn't enough simply to be aware of feelings: you also need to respond appropriately and skilfully. Let's begin with how you manage your own emotions.

People who are emotionally intelligent are able to control what they do with their emotions. They can choose wisely whether to state assertively what they are experiencing or to maintain a poker-faced silence. Suppose, for example, that you notice you are becoming angry in a conversation with another person. In some situations it might be important and useful to disclose that you're feeling angry, perhaps going on to explore with the other person what's led up to this and what needs to happen now. In other contexts it might be unhelpful or pointless to reveal that you're angry. As Aristotle wrote, to be angry with the right person, to the right degree, isn't easy.

Here are two simple ideas which can be helpful. The first is simply to count to ten before you respond to something which has triggered a strong emotion in you. The second is to take yourself out of a situation where you sense that you may be about to respond inappropriately, giving yourself time to calm down, to consider what you want and to decide what, if anything, to do.

Relationship management

Likewise, as you become aware of how the other person is feeling, you need to choose how to respond. An emotionally intelligent person has a range of social skills that enables him or her to respond appropriately and successfully to a wide range of people and situations. For example, imagine you are talking to someone and you realize he has become bored. If the conversation is important, you may need to persist but change how you're engaging with him so that you regain his interest. At other times, it might be more appropriate to recognize that the other person isn't interested in what you're saying and simply end the conversation. Being flexible in how you respond is valuable.

A very useful skill in responding from your empathic understanding of the other person is the ability to play back what you've heard or noticed. When people hear their situation played back accurately, they feel understood, and may well feel valued. This helps to build rapport and enhances the relationship between you.

Understanding what motivates you

I'd like to explore the idea of self-awareness in a little more detail since this is the foundation for managing yourself and your relationships with other people. It is worth spending some time – on your own or in conversation with someone you trust – to explore important questions such as:

- What are my values?
- What are my beliefs about people, including myself?
- What are my goals, both short term and long term?

It is also worth examining your self-talk, which refers to the things that you say to yourself, inside your head as it were. The basis of a cognitive behavioural approach to personal change can be summed up in the words of an ancient Stoic philosopher, Epictetus, who wrote that 'People are disturbed not by things, but by the views which they take of them.' In other words, what you think about a situation shapes how you feel and behave. For example, compare the likely impact of this pair of statements:

- The world should be fair.
- It's important to me that I treat others fairly.

The second statement is more realistic than the first. Similarly, the second statement below is less sweeping and more likely to be helpful:

- I'm useless at interviews.
- I perform better at interviews when I prepare thoroughly.

So, consider the messages that you say to yourself and how this self-talk affects your responses to events. Maybe there are things that you believe or tell yourself that are neither true nor helpful. Identify too what would be more useful self-talk.

Exercise 2.2 What motivates you?

Make some notes in response to these questions:

- What are your values?
- What are your beliefs about people, including yourself?
- What are your goals, both short term and long term?
- What unhelpful things do you say to yourself?
- What would be more useful alternative things to say to yourself?

Developing your emotional intelligence

A survey of managers in a UK supermarket chain found that those with high emotional intelligence experienced less stress, enjoyed better health, performed better and reported a better work–life balance. There are wide-reaching benefits – both for yourself and for those around you – in being more emotionally intelligent.

Whereas conventional intelligence – as measured by IQ – is more or less given, you can improve your emotional intelligence as you go through life. Your life experiences – and how you handle them – will be a rich source of opportunities to develop your EQ, as it's sometimes called.

Here are some ways in which you might use your day-to-day experiences to develop each of the four quadrants of the emotional intelligence framework set out earlier in the chapter. Choose those that you think will be helpful for you personally.

Self-awareness

- Develop the habit of noticing and putting a name to your feelings. Regularly take a moment to check inwardly how you're feeling, and then complete a three-word sentence that begins 'I feel . . .'
- Spend some time working through Exercise 2.2 to clarify what really matters to you in your life.

Empathy

- Develop your active listening skills, listening to understand how the world looks from the perspective of the other person. Ask open questions that invite others to tell you more about what matters to them. Observe their body language, listening for the things that may be important but are not being said. Try to pick up on the emotions as well as the facts.
- Who are the key people that you interact with at home and at work? What really matters to each of these people? What support do they need from you?

Self-management

- Note what happens next time you are in a conflict situation. Do you passively withdraw or give up? Do you aggressively seek to win at the expense of the other party? Or do you assertively look for how both of you can gain some benefit – a win–win outcome?
- Observe those people who leave you feeling drained or upset or somehow less positive. What do they do that triggers this? How do you collude with them? What can you do to reduce the time you spend with them?

Relationship management

- Observe those people who create positive, nourishing relationships with other people. What can you learn from how they interact with people?
- Keep a journal that records significant events where you felt strongly about something or someone. Make a note of how you felt, what you thought, what you said or did, what you didn't say or do, and what the consequences were. From time to time look back at your journal and see if there are any patterns.

Exercise 2.3 Developing your emotional intelligence

Choose two or three of these ideas on developing your emotional intelligence and try them out. Notice and reflect upon what happens.

3

Understanding your personality type

Introduction

In this chapter we will look at a number of aspects of personality. As we explored in the previous chapter, self-awareness and understanding other people can help you to manage yourself and your relationship more successfully.

The most widely used personality questionnaire in the world is the Myers-Briggs Type Indicator®. The MBTI® was developed by two Americans, Katharine Briggs and her daughter, Isabel Briggs Myers, based on the psychological theories of Carl Jung. The questionnaire is a self-report instrument – that is, respondents answer a number of questions about themselves. The underlying model proposes that each of us has an innate preference on four separate dimensions of personality. In her book *Introduction to Type* Isabel Myers summarizes these four dimensions as in Table 3.1.

This leads to a four-letter description of an individual's personality type – for instance, INTP or ESFJ. There are 16 possible combinations, and the way in which the different dimensions of the MBTI® combine is significant. In this chapter we will simply look at the four dimensions separately and won't explore how the various dimensions interact with one another.

The Extravert–Introvert dimension

These two words – Extravert and Introvert – were coined originally by Carl Jung and have now entered everyday language, albeit not exactly as defined originally by Jung. The thesaurus on my laptop suggests that an 'extrovert' – it doesn't contain 'extravert' – is an outgoing or gregarious person while an 'introvert' is a shy person.

In the MBTI® the Extravert–Introvert dimension refers to where you get your energy from and where you prefer to focus your

Table 3.1 Dimensions of the Myers-Briggs Type Indicator®

Extraversion (E) People who prefer Extraversion like to focus on the outer world of people and activity.	*Introversion (I)* People who prefer Introversion like to focus on their own inner world of ideas and experiences.
Sensing (S) People who prefer Sensing like to take in information that is real and tangible – what is actually happening.	*Intuition (N)* People who prefer Intuition like to take in information by seeing the big picture, focusing on the relationships and connections between facts.
Thinking (T) People who prefer to use Thinking in decision-making like to look at the logical consequences of a choice or action.	*Feeling (F)* People who prefer to use Feeling in decision-making like to consider what is important to them and to others involved.
Judging (J) People who use their Judging process in the outer world like to live in a planned, orderly way, seeking to regulate and manage their lives.	*Perceiving (P)* People who prefer to use their Perceiving process in the outer world like to live in a flexible, spontaneous way, seeking to experience and understand life, rather than control it.

attention. Extraverts are energized by being with other people whereas Introverts recharge their batteries, so to speak, by withdrawing into their inner world. As an illustration, returning after a busy day at work to find a party going on at home, an Extravert is likely to feel energized whereas an Introvert would rather have a quiet soak in the bath.

Jung, Myers and Briggs state that each of the dimensions is one of Type rather than Trait. Each of us is born – they claim – as either an Extravert or an Introvert. To illustrate this notion of Type, take a sheet of paper and write your usual signature. You probably do this quite naturally without thinking about it. Now write your signature again with your other hand. You are likely to find that this feels unnatural or awkward and requires you to think about what you're doing. Writing with your non-preferred hand takes more effort. If you broke your wrist and had to use this other hand for some time, you'd find it becomes easier though probably never as comfortable as with your preferred hand.

In days gone by, people who were naturally left-handed were often forced at school to write with their right hand. MBTI® theory recognizes that, through life experiences such as your upbringing or schooling or employment, you may develop facility with the other dimension, but this will require more effort than using your innate and natural preference.

I myself don't agree that each of the dimensions is one of Type rather than Trait. I think that people fall on some kind of continuum – perhaps a statistically normal distribution – from extremely gregarious Extraverts to folk somewhere in the middle to those who are very shy and Introverted.

Myers and Briggs are not claiming that preference on any of the dimensions is necessarily an indicator of ability. There are some highly socially skilled Introverts and some emotionally unintelligent Extraverts, for instance. But Introverts will find it takes more energy to interact with others than Extraverts do. As an illustration, I have a strong natural preference for Introvert. In my work, however, I frequently facilitate workshops where I need to engage in a lot of Extravert-style behaviour. I feel more tired at the end of a workshop than if I were naturally more Extraverted. I hope, however, that I have learnt to carry out these behaviours well.

One way of caricaturing Extraverts and Introverts is that Extraverts speak first and maybe think later, whereas Introverts think first and maybe speak later. I once had an Extravert boss who frequently thought out loud. It took me some time to realize that he didn't expect me to carry out all of the ideas he was talking about as he developed his views by vocalizing them. An Introvert is likely to agree with the maxim: 'If you have nothing to say then say nothing.' On the other hand, I knew one Extraverted director who reckoned that if you have nothing to say then it's important to say it eloquently. His serious point here was that in some meetings it's important to be seen as a player and you need to make a contribution early on. And, unless you say something ridiculous, it probably doesn't matter what you say so long as you appear confident.

In my work as a coach with individuals, I find that I introduce the Extravert–Introvert dimension mainly with Introverts and only occasionally with Extraverts. Being aware of their natural preference can enable some Introverts to modify their behaviour in meetings, for example. They may recognize that if they wait till they have fully thought through their position then the meeting will have moved on to another item and they will have lost the chance to contribute. Hence they see the need to speak up sooner and more frequently in some situations. I myself use a couple of tactics to counter my own Introvert preference. I will, for example, signpost that I have a contribution to make by saying something along the lines of 'There are two points I'd like to make here.' Or I give myself permission to come out with something that isn't fully worked out by saying things such as 'I'd like to think out loud for a minute' or 'Let me play devil's advocate.'

As with the other dimensions of the MBTI®, the model enables you both to understand your own behaviour and to appreciate how other people behave. So, for example, an Extraverted team leader may see the need consciously to create opportunities in team meetings for the more Introverted people – or perhaps those who are less experienced or confident – to contribute their ideas. Awareness of the preferences of yourself and others on the Extravert–Introvert dimension can help you to communicate and manage relationships more effectively.

Exercise 3.1 Extravert or Introvert?

Read through the descriptions of the Extravert and Introvert preferences and consider where you sit on this dimension. Do you have a strong preference for either end of the spectrum, or do you see yourself somewhere in the middle? Note that the theory suggests that you have an innate preference for one or the other, though your past experiences or the demands of your role may mean that you behave in ways that aren't your natural preference.

Think too of some individuals in your private or professional life. Which of these show a clear preference for Extraversion or Introversion?

The Sensing–Intuition dimension

The Sensing–Intuition dimension refers to how people prefer to take in information and what kind of information they like to pay attention to. The words 'Sensing' and 'Intuition' may be misleading, and I prefer to talk about an S preference or an N preference. Note that N rather than I is used since Myers and Briggs use I to refer to Introversion.

People with an S preference like to see the detail and want information to be precise and accurate. When they look around a room they are likely to notice and remember lots of specific details of the items in the room. They focus on what is concrete, and are likely to value doing things as they were done before if this worked well.

However, people with an N preference are happy with the big picture only, and may get bored if you give them too much detail. They may be more interested in patterns and meanings, and enjoy exploring possibilities. They may well value the abstract and theoretical rather than the concrete and practical. They like to do things in new ways, even if the old way worked well.

Awareness of your own and others' preferences on the S–N dimension is very useful in communicating effectively. If your boss has an S preference, for example, you are likely to have to provide lots of detailed information when making a proposal. However, if your boss has an N preference, then you may be more influential if you describe the big picture and highlight the possibilities.

Exercise 3.2 S or N preference?

Think about how you like to take in information. Do you have a strong S preference, valuing lots of detail and what is real and tangible? Do you have a strong N preference for the big picture, patterns and possibilities? Or do you see yourself somewhere in the middle?

Think too of some individuals that you need to communicate with regularly. Who shows a strong preference for S or N? How can you best pass on information and ideas to them?

The Thinking–Feeling dimension

The third dimension of the MBTI® reflects how people prefer to make decisions. Those with a Thinking or T preference use logic and analysis to work out what to do. They are able to take a detached standpoint and apply objective criteria or rules or principles to make a decision. They seek to understand cause and effect, or to weigh up costs and benefits. They like to be consistent in their decision-making. They may also be good at spotting the flaws in the logic of other people's proposals. At work they are likely to be task focused.

People at the other end of this continuum with a Feeling or F preference base their decisions on their values and convictions. They seem to be in the middle of the situation, focusing on how decisions will affect everyone involved. They seek to establish common ground, and hope to create harmony. They like to treat people as individuals, and fairness is more important than consistency. At work they may emphasize people rather than task.

As with the other dimensions, it can be useful to utilize both perspectives to make even better decisions. For example, in situations of organizational change, such as the merger of two departments, a T approach is useful in working out what will be a highly effective structure, while a more consultative F approach is needed to ensure that the people affected are treated with fairness and respect and hence are more likely to buy into the change.

Exercise 3.3 *T or F preference?*

Think about occasions when you've made important decisions that had an impact on other people. Did you analyse the situation logically, identifying the pros and cons of different options? Or did you attempt to find a way forward that appealed to everyone involved?

The Judging–Perceiving dimension

The dimension of MBTI® which I use most frequently with coaching clients after Extravert–Introvert is the fourth and final dimension, namely Judging–Perceiving. The words 'Judging' and 'Perceiving' may give a misleading impression – this dimension isn't really about judgement or perception. Hence, it is often preferable to speak about a J preference and a P preference.

People with a J preference like to operate in a planned and orderly way. Faced with a task, they are likely to make a plan with milestones and deadlines. They may even create a contingency plan in case things don't quite work out with their original plan. They hate last-minute changes, and may become stressed by undue time pressure.

People with a P preference, on the other hand, like to keep options open and are comfortable simply going with the flow. When deadlines loom they are energized by last-minute time pressures. They feel constrained by plans and dislike making a decision until they have to.

Once again I think that this dimension is a continuum rather than an either/or Type preference. I myself have a P preference, but it took me several years to be confident that my self-assessment was accurate and I think I am nearer the middle on this continuum. I have worked with colleagues who had an incredibly strong P preference, which I found frustrating at times. I have also worked with people whose strong J preference for planning in great detail struck me as pedantic and excessive. As my own confessions might indicate, differences on this dimension may well lead to conflict.

Because of the complexity of life in modern organizations, people with a P preference often need to learn to work in a J style. For example, I learnt through experience in my early years in management development that if I wanted to run a course then I needed to arrange things well in advance by, for instance, booking a venue and calling for nominations to the programme. But my ability to work in a J style is a learnt behaviour, and you would be foolish, for example, to ask me to project manage the construction of a new office block. I can manage a timeline, but Gantt charts are just too detailed for my liking! This reflects both my P preference and also, as we considered above, my N preference.

Exercise 3.4 J or P preference?

Imagine that you are embarking on a project in either your professional or private life. Do you like to make a detailed plan with milestones? Or do you prefer to start off and work out what you need to do as you go along? To what extent do your preferences change in your private life compared to your professional life?

Think of some people that you need to collaborate with. Which of these have a preference on the J–P dimension that is very different from your own? What do you need to do to co-operate effectively with them?

Type Dynamics

The four dimensions explored above lead to a four-letter description of an individual's personality type – for instance, my own Type preference is INTP. There are 16 possible combinations, and the way in which the different dimensions of the MBTI® combine is significant. In this chapter we have simply looked at the four dimensions separately and haven't explored how the various dimensions interact with one another. If you'd like to know more about this, a topic which is known as Type Dynamics, you might look at *Introduction to Type Dynamics and Development* by Katharine Myers and Linda Kirby.

If you are interested in using the MBTI® professionally, you need to be qualified to administer it. You can find out about training workshops to become qualified from the website of the business psychology consultancy OPP – see <www.opp.eu.com>.

Awareness and responsibility

In the opening chapter we noted that one way of using the ideas in this book is, first, to consider how your awareness shifts as you reflect on the ideas and, second, to choose how you will behave differently in response to your raised awareness. The four dimensions of the MBTI® are useful both in understanding and managing yourself and also in appreciating others and how you need to interact with them. In trying to understand other people, you inevitably have to make a judgement on their preferences on the dimensions of the MBTI® and it can often be difficult to get this correct. Nevertheless, knowledge of your own Type and an appreciation of the preferences of the other person can help you to communicate more effectively, to improve relationships, to be more assertive, to manage others well, and to influence more successfully.

As an illustration, let's revisit the topic of emotional intelligence, which we considered in the previous chapter. If you have an F rather than a T preference, you will more naturally consider the impact of change on other people, and you are likely to seek harmony when making a decision. Hence you need also to consider whether you are avoiding making tough but necessary choices, and perhaps force yourself to make a decision that feels unpleasant to you. On the other hand, if you have a T preference, your natural tendency will be to analyse the various factors in the situation and make a decision which is logical based on your analysis. You may need to make a conscious effort to consider what the various other people in the situation need, fear or hope for, and take their feelings into account as well as your own logical assessment of the facts of the matter.

To return to an example mentioned earlier, if your manager has an S preference, which means he values detail, then it will be important when putting forward an idea to give him the kind of detail that he requires – and maybe lots of it. However, if your boss has an N preference, then she may be bored by the detail and you need to give her an overview which sets out the future possibilities that your idea opens up.

Awareness – of your own and of others' preferences – coupled with a suitable response which reflects this awareness is more likely to lead to success.

4

Ideas from Transactional Analysis

Introduction

In this chapter I'd like to explore a number of ideas from Transactional Analysis that can help you to manage yourself and your relationships with other people.

TA – as it is often called – is a psychological theory that seeks to explain how individuals think, feel, behave and interact with others, often in patterns that are repeated through life. It is a way of understanding what happens within and between people. TA is fundamentally a psychoanalytic approach which assumes that our early childhood experiences profoundly shape – generally unconsciously – how we live our lives.

However, it is possible to use ideas from TA at a cognitive level. The models set out in this chapter may increase your awareness as you view things and make sense of your situation from a new perspective. And, when you begin to think differently about your situation you may then go on to respond or act differently. In this way TA can also be regarded as a cognitive behavioural approach which can help you to think and behave more effectively.

The first model that we shall look at is the notion of Parent, Adult and Child ego states. I reckon that I sketch this model with a coaching client perhaps once a week. In my experience, people not only find it easy to understand but also – and more importantly – find that it offers a useful way of looking at how they are interacting with other people.

Ego states

We develop our personality as we go through life, but much of it is shaped by our experiences in early childhood. Some aspects – our

Child ego state – are like replays of how we ourselves behaved as young children seeking the love or approval of powerful figures in our lives, such as parents, older siblings or teachers. Other aspects of our personality – our **Parent ego state** – are based on feelings, attitudes and behaviours that we copied – or swallowed whole, as it were – from our parents or other authority figures. As we grow up we also integrate our experiences of healthy, co-operative relationships and of times when we coped well with difficulties – these emotional memories form our **Adult ego state**. Each of us spends time in and switches between these three psychological states – Parent, Adult and Child.

The Child and Parent ego states are subdivided in Transactional Analysis. When you were a young child you often had to adapt to the demands of your parents or carers. You may have learnt to be polite to others, or to be quiet when your mother or father was in a certain mood. You may have learnt that certain emotions were acceptable, but that it wasn't all right to show anger or to cry. Later in life, when you are acting on the basis of these historic and often by now unconscious memories, you are in your **Adapted Child ego state**.

However, when you were three or four years old you also spent time laughing, splashing water, playing with paint or glue or sand, and running around. When you are older you might revert to these times, and you are then in your **Free Child ego state**.

If you find yourself in a conversation wagging your finger at the other person, speaking in a harsh tone, pointing out what he has done wrong and telling him how he should have behaved, then almost certainly you are in a **Critical Parent ego state**. This illustrates how when people are in a particular ego state their thoughts, feelings, words and body language are generally consistent with one another.

However, when you were a young child your parents also looked after you and ensured that you were safe and well. Perhaps they took your hand and explained that it was important to wait for the green man to appear on the traffic signal before crossing the road. When you find yourself years later looking to protect and look after one of your friends or colleagues, then you may well have gone into a **Nurturing Parent ego state**. One thing that both

Critical Parent and Nurturing Parent ego states have in common is that both are about controlling the other person.

The Adult ego state is not usually subdivided within TA. Hence, there are five possible ego states – Critical Parent, Nurturing Parent, Adapted Child, Free Child and Adult – represented in Figure 4.1.

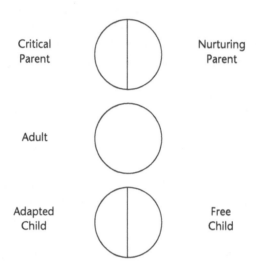

Critical Parent

Nurturing Parent

Adult

Adapted Child

Free Child

Figure 4.1 Ego states

Being in an Adult ego state – focused on the here and now, look-ing to collaborate with others and to solve problems, thinking logically and aware of your own and other people's emotions – is generally a very resourceful state to operate from. However, there are times when it is valuable to be in one of the other ego states, and each of these can be divided further into positive or negative behaviours. So, for example:

- Good table manners reflect a positive aspect of Adapted Child, while sulking is a negative manifestation.
- Being in Free Child is very useful at a party or when brain-storming creative ideas, but is inappropriate when driving on a motorway.

- Pointing out to someone that her behaviour is dangerous might reflect a positive version of Critical Parent, but losing your temper when a friend makes a small mistake is negative.
- Offering to help a hard-pressed colleague is positive, whereas not letting your 17-year-old daughter stay out after ten o'clock may be a smothering and negative version of Nurturing Parent.

Exercise 4.1 Egograms

Each of us spends time in all five of these ego states. Think back over a typical week. In your notebook, write down five numbers adding up to 100 that represent the percentage of your time that you spend in:

- Critical Parent
- Nurturing Parent
- Adult
- Adapted Child
- Free Child.

You may find it useful to create two sets of numbers that reflect how you are when at work and how you are when not at work.

- Which ego state would you like to spend more time in?
- Which ego state would you like to spend less time in?
- What will you do to make these changes?

Transactions

So far, in considering ego states, we have been concerned with the processes within an individual person. Transactional Analysis – as the name implies – is concerned with the communications or transactions between people and the relationships thereby created. When I say something to you and you reply, this is a transaction. Transactions – a stimulus plus a response – are the building blocks of communication.

One of the things which can happen in relationships is that we establish typical ways of interacting with one another. For example, a manager with a very directive, command and control style of managing will frequently be operating from a Critical Parent ego state. This may well engender Adapted Child responses from those who work for him. The typical pattern of interaction between this manager and a subordinate is Critical Parent–Adapted Child (see Figure 4.2). (Note that even the word 'subordinate' – rather than, for example, 'team member' or 'colleague' – in the last sentence suggests a certain type of relationship.)

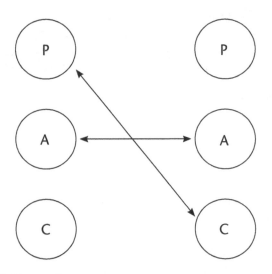

Figure 4.2 Transactions

In *Turning to One Another* Meg Wheatley writes that, 'Those who act superior can't help but treat others as objects to accomplish their causes and plans.' If this way of interacting becomes the norm, then the culture becomes one characterized by Parent–Child behaviour. This can be quite effective – it is the basis of traditional military discipline, for instance. And it may suit all parties. It gives superiors a sense of power, control, status and prestige. It offers subordinates a sense that their role is to follow orders or instructions, which can be quite comfortable. However, it means that the group isn't drawing on many of the ideas and resources of its members, and they in turn may be feeling less motivated and gaining less satisfaction.

Generally an Adult–Adult relationship is more likely to be healthy and productive. To engage in an Adult–Adult conversation, you need to be straight in your communication and regard the other person as your equal simply because he or she is another human being (even though you may be more senior, experienced or talented). This is the basis of assertive communication.

The key to breaking a pattern of unhelpful Parent–Child transactions is to consistently communicate from an Adult ego state and to continually invite the other party to operate from his or her Adult. Note that there is no guarantee that the other party will respond from Adult – all you can do is to remain in Adult yourself and keep inviting an Adult response. Changing such an established pattern of interactions may well be difficult, not least because it requires the other party to change his or her behaviour too.

So, for example, you may realize that in your interactions with your manager you are coming from an Adapted Child ego state in response to his Critical Parent. With this awareness, you may attempt to remain in Adult whenever you meet your manager, inviting an Adult response. Alternatively, you might be a manager becoming frustrated by the seeming inability or unwillingness of one of your team to take appropriate responsibility. His Adapted Child behaviour is hooking your Critical Parent. You might seek then to remain in Adult, continually inviting him to take more responsibility and operate from his own Adult ego state.

The idea of ego states is also very helpful in situations where someone is behaving passively when he or she would prefer to be assertive. When someone is acting passively, it will often be the case that this person is in an Adapted Child ego state. Seeking to create Adult–Adult transactions is a useful way of behaving assertively. We shall look at this in more detail in Chapter 6 on assertiveness and handling conflict.

Exercise 4.2 Analysing transactions

Identify a relationship which you have with a relative, friend, acquaintance or work colleague that is to some extent problematic. Think about how you and the other person typically interact, or perhaps interact when things go wrong. How would you describe the pattern of transactions between the two of you? What might you do differently to make it more likely that these will be Adult–Adult transactions?

Scripts, positions and drivers

Another idea from Transactional Analysis is the notion of life script. Eric Berne, the founder of TA, maintained that each of us early in childhood decides upon a plan for our life, our life script. This is influenced by our parents and our early environment, but it is also a decision that each of us makes. The decisions we make in early childhood are not through the kind of deliberate thinking that we might use later in life. Rather, they are emotional decisions we make in response to external pressures as a way of surviving and having our needs met in a world that is often perceived by an infant as hostile.

These early childhood experiences and decisions mean that we end up following a life script such as:

- I mustn't be me (which might manifest itself in feelings of inferiority);
- I mustn't be a child (which might inhibit someone from being playful, having fun or behaving spontaneously);
- I mustn't do anything (which might lead to over-cautiousness and inability to make decisions).

Note that the life script planned by the individual as an infant is not necessarily the same as that person's life story. What actually happens will be affected by decisions the individual makes as an adult, including decisions for change that he or she may make through coaching or counselling. As the examples indicate, to explore a life script in depth may mean working at a psychodynamic level with someone who is trained and competent to work in this way.

An idea that arises from life scripts is the notion of life positions. There are four life positions which are based on how you see the essential value in yourself and in others:

- **I'm OK, you're OK.** This is a *healthy* position, where you feel good about yourself and others, seek to collaborate and find it comfortable to behave assertively.
- **I'm not OK, you're OK.** This is a *depressive* position where you feel one down on others and tend to behave passively.

- **I'm OK, you're not OK.** This is a *defensive* position where you feel one up on others but behave aggressively, competitively or insensitively to justify your stance.
- **I'm not OK, you're not OK.** This is a *futile* position where you consider that neither you nor others are any good and often feel hopeless and helpless.

An idea that is related to the notion of life script and that can be explored at a less intense level is the concept of drivers. As an illustration, you can consider and address an issue such as perfectionism in terms of having a driver to 'be perfect', a habitual way of behaving that has been shaped by your upbringing or childhood experiences. Five common drivers are:

- Be perfect.
- Be strong.
- Try hard.
- Please others.
- Hurry up.

If you become aware that your typical way of behaving is based on one of these drivers, you then have greater choice over how to conduct yourself. You can utilize the strengths of your driver when this is appropriate, and you can choose to respond differently when it isn't – in other words, you needn't be ruled by your driver.

Games and the drama triangle

Another useful concept in Transactional Analysis is the idea that people play **games**. A game is a repetitive pattern of transactions between people where something is happening out of awareness at a psychological level that is different from what is taking place at a surface level and which leads to some kind of outcome or pay-off, generally but not always in the form of negative feelings or attitudes. In playing a psychological game we are following outdated strategies that we used as children to get what we needed. Game-playing is one way of manifesting and reinforcing a life script.

When we are caught up in a psychological game, the presence of negative feelings may provide a clue that things aren't quite as they appear to be. There may be hidden meanings behind what's said, and communications aren't entirely straight.

TA writers often give catchy names to games. For example, in a game called 'If It Weren't For You', a mother tells her children repeatedly how she longs to travel overseas but can't because she has to look after them. However, even when her children are grown up she still finds reasons not to make those foreign trips. Or, in a common game called 'Yes, But . . .', the player repeatedly seeks advice but always finds reasons not to accept it. Such a player might interact with a partner who himself is playing the game of 'Why Don't You?' in which he continually makes suggestions that are rejected.

Exercise 4.3 Drivers, scripts and games

- Which of the four life positions do you think you yourself take?
- Which of the five drivers do you recognize in yourself?
- What psychological games do you engage in? With whom?

Think now of one or two people that you interact with frequently. For each person:

- Which life position does this person take?
- Which drivers shape his or her behaviour?
- What psychological games does he or she play? How are you involved in these games?

Stephen Karpman devised a framework for analysing games, the **drama triangle** (see Figure 4.3). The three roles in the drama triangle are Persecutor, Victim and Rescuer. The **Persecutor** puts others down, and is coming from a life position of 'I'm OK, you're not OK'. The **Victim** sees him- or herself as one down, and is coming from 'I'm not OK, you're OK'. The **Rescuer** also sees the Victim as one down but responds by offering help. When people play games they are in one of these three inauthentic roles, using old strategies in Parent or Child ego states rather than responding in the here and now from an Adult ego state.

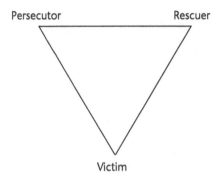

Figure 4.3 The drama triangle

In the drama triangle, the Victim may seek out a Persecutor to put him down or a Rescuer to confirm his belief that he can't cope on his own. The drama triangle often involves a switch in roles as it is played out. For example, imagine a situation where a woman (the Victim) is married to a husband (the Persecutor) who abuses her, either physically or emotionally. For a while she copes with this by endlessly complaining to a friend (the Rescuer) who spends hours listening and offering suggestions that are never taken up. There are various ways in which a switch might occur. The woman might start an affair with another man, moving from Victim to Persecutor while her husband now becomes the Victim. Or her friend might lose her patience and her temper one day, switching from Rescuer to Persecutor.

One way of dealing with game-playing is to step out of the drama triangle and respond authentically from an Adult ego state or from one of the positive versions of the other ego states. The **winner's triangle** is an alternative to the drama triangle which recognizes that people may genuinely be vulnerable, that others really do have power or potency, and that helpers can be a useful resource to support others (Figure 4.4 overleaf).

In their chapter in *The Complete Handbook of Coaching* Trudi Newton and Rosemary Napper write that

The clue to moving from game playing to authenticity is to recognize the truth behind the game roles: people do have real

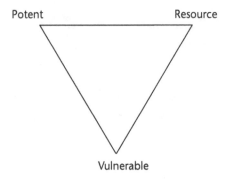

Figure 4.4 The winner's triangle

problems for which they have not yet learned the strategies to solve; people are genuinely and appropriately concerned about others' welfare and can offer support without taking over; and people can be assertive about what they can and cannot do without 'pushing' or blaming others.

Exercise 4.4 The drama triangle

Think of someone you know who frequently finds him- or herself in Victim mode.

- What role do you take in response?
- What might you do to move from the drama triangle to the winner's triangle?

5

Conversations

Introduction

Relationships are built on conversations. The conversations you have – and the conversations you avoid having – shape the nature of your relationships with those around you. The ability to engage in the conversations that matter lies at the heart of creating effective relationships. If you are a manager, then the conversations you have with the people who work for you are vital to how well you work together.

In this chapter we shall first look at four key skills of conversation – listening, playing back, questioning and voicing. These conversational skills are invaluable if you wish to behave assertively or handle conflict constructively, which are topics explored in the next chapter. We end by considering how you might handle difficult conversations.

Levels of listening

In her book *Turning to One Another* Meg Wheatley writes: 'Why is being heard so healing? I don't know the full answer to that question, but I do know that it has something to do with the fact that listening creates relationship.' I think this is a tremendously important point. Simply listening to another person nurtures the relationship between you.

There are different types of listening, illustrated in the ladder of listening in Figure 5.1. First, and this is a very common form of listening in many contexts, is **not listening at all**. I know one woman who describes her husband's style of listening as 'listening while watching Sky Sports'.

A second way is **listening, waiting to speak**. This is when I want to talk and will wait for as short a time as possible before starting to speak. Sometimes I might wait for you to pause, but equally I might interrupt you in mid-sentence. In a social situation, swapping news and stories, this type of listening is common.

A third way of listening – and it is typical of the kind of listening that goes on in many meetings – is **listening to disagree**. I want my point of view to prevail or to get my way. I'm listening for the weak points in what you say, and when I spot one I pounce. In some situations – in Parliament, in a court of law or in much academic discourse – this is the normal form of conversation, and it may be entirely appropriate. It is about debate and argument. It is about winning and losing, or perhaps compromising. And some of the language we use to describe this form of conversation reveals its essentially adversarial nature:

- I attack your position.
- I defend my views.
- I overcome your reservations.
- I probe for the weak points in your argument.
- I win the case.
- I lose the argument.

A fourth type of listening – and this way of listening is vital in developing deep relationships – is **listening to understand**. This is the level of listening needed to coach well. In listening to understand, I am trying to see the world as it appears through your eyes. I am trying to appreciate what you're thinking and how you're feeling. I want to understand your dreams and your hopes, your fears and your doubts. The word that is often used here is 'empathy'. Note that when you understand someone's point of view, this doesn't necessarily mean that you agree with it.

Exercise 5.1 How do you listen?

Over the next few days monitor the quality of your own listening when you are in conversation with others. Notice how it varies in different situations or when you are with different people.

- When do you not listen?
- When do you listen, waiting to speak?
- When do you listen to disagree?
- When do you listen to understand?

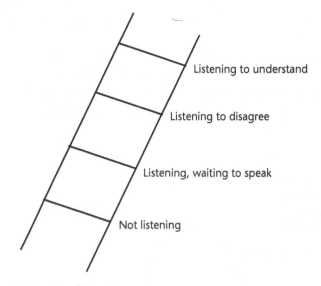

Figure 5.1 Levels of listening

Listening with the head, the heart and the gut

Another model to illustrate different ways of listening uses the metaphors of listening with the head, the heart and the gut.

Listening with your head means focusing on the words that the other person actually says. At a thinking level, she is communicating facts, information, arguments, ideas and concepts. You might imagine that she is communicating from her head to your head, and you may speak back from your head to her head.

However, people communicate at a feelings level too. They may vocalize their feelings – 'I'm angry', 'I feel sad', 'This is so exciting', and so on. Often, however, the words spoken may be only the tip of the iceberg and the feelings that lie beneath the words may be expressed non-verbally – through tone of voice, or body language, or facial expression. To listen effectively you need to tune into what is not being said. You might call listening at a feelings level **listening with your heart**.

At a deeper level still, you might **listen with your gut** – that is, with your intuition – and pick up messages that are there but again are not spoken. Sometimes your gut tells you things well before your intellect catches on. With your gut, you might hear about the other person's fears or hopes or needs.

Figure 5.2 illustrates these three levels of listening using an analogy with an iceberg. Above the surface you pick up with your head the words that are actually said. Below the surface you pick up with your heart and your gut what is not said – the emotions, fears, hopes, and so on.

With your head you hear:

What is actually said:

- Words
- Facts
- Information
- Task
- Formal agenda

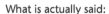

With your heart and with your gut you hear:

What is not said:

- Intentions
- Motivations
- Needs
- Fears
- Aspirations
- Power struggles
- Informal agenda

Figure 5.2 Listening with the head, the heart and the gut

Playing back

The second conversational skill, which is an excellent way of showing the other person that you have been listening to him, is to play back your understanding of what he's said or perhaps what he's communicated non-verbally through his body language, facial expression or tone of voice. In a coaching context I use three main ways of playing back to the client my understanding of what he or she has said.

First, I will **summarize** to play back my understanding of the key points. I might, for instance, say something like 'You seem to be saying that there are three issues here . . .' I will often use a summary to cover an extended piece of conversation.

Second, I will **paraphrase** what the person has said. For instance, the other person might say, 'It feels like I'm banging my head against a brick wall', and I might respond with 'It sounds like you're feeling very frustrated and perhaps a bit angry.' There are times when it's useful for someone to hear her words played back in a different formulation, but a risk in paraphrasing is that you distort their meaning so that your playback is unhelpful.

Third, I will **reflect back** to the person what he has said, repeating his exact words. Sometimes there is energy or significance in the precise words or metaphors that someone uses, and it can be powerful to stay with his exact language. In the previous illustration, for example, I might respond with 'Tell me more about what it's like to be banging your head against a brick wall.' Or sometimes there might be a single word that seems pregnant with significance, perhaps indicated by the person's tone of voice.

I find that playing back your understanding is a very useful way of managing a conversation. It helps to check or modify your understanding of the other person's position. Moreover, when people feel that they have been heard and understood, they are likely to be ready to move on in the conversation. Playing back also gives you time to think about where to go next in the conversation, which can be very useful when you are coaching or negotiating.

Questioning

The third conversational skill is the ability to ask open questions that invite the other person to explore or explain his position in some detail. In coaching, for example, a good question is one that helps the individual to think.

It is very useful to distinguish between open and closed questions. As an illustration, consider the difference between the closed question 'Did you like the film?' and the open question 'What did you like about the film?' The latter is likely to generate far more information.

Open questions usually begin with Kipling's trusted friends:

> I keep six honest serving-men
> (They taught me all I knew);
> Their names are *What* and *Why* and *When*
> And *How* and *Where* and *Who*.

A word of caution about asking a question beginning with 'Why?' This can often come across as unduly challenging and might provoke defensiveness in the other person, who may feel forced to justify his or her views. It is easy to soften a 'Why?' question by saying something like 'I'm interested in what led you to do that' or 'What is your intention in doing this?' Note too that these questions are more focused than a simple 'Why?' question – the first example is backward looking and the second example is forward looking.

Closed questions, interestingly, generally begin with a verb:

- Have you...?
- Are you...?
- Could you...?
- Will you...?

Occasionally, a closed question is just what is called for. For instance, you may want to check out whether someone really is committed to an action by asking a question such as: 'So, will you speak to him tonight?'

I also think that the best questions are short, and the word I like to use in this regard is 'crisp'. A crisp question – simply expressed – invites the other person to focus on the most important issue.

Exercise 5.2 What kind of questions do you ask?

Consider the questions that you ask. In particular, notice whether you tend to ask closed questions that can be answered with one word or open questions that invite a fuller answer.

Notice too how many words it takes you to ask a question. It is often possible to ask a helpful, crisp question in half a dozen words, or fewer: 'What's your view?'

One other thing to pay attention to is whether you ask leading questions. A leading question is one which already contains the answer or at least a suggested answer. It is often advice disguised as a question. For example:

- Don't you think it's time to end that relationship?
- Would it be a good idea to sell the car?

In my view, if you have a suggestion to make then it's better simply to state this. Here are alternative formulations of these leading questions, paired with an open question seeking the views of the other person:

- I believe it's time for you to end that relationship. What do you think?
- I think it would it be a good idea to sell the car. What are your thoughts?

Voicing

The fourth conversational skill is voicing – the ability to state clearly what you think and the reasons that underlie your thinking.

There is a place for small talk and polite conversation. When you meet someone for the first time at a party, for instance, it is normal to talk about your journey or the weather or how you know the host. Such small talk may be the first step to a much more meaningful level of engagement. However, it may be important to go beyond polite talk and speak authentically. In *Difficult Conversations* Douglas Stone, Bruce Patton and Sheila Heen write that:

When we fail to share what's important to us, we detach ourselves from others and damage our relationships.

A relationship takes hold and grows when both participants experience themselves and the other as being authentic.

It can be both helpful and powerful not merely to state your point of view but also to reveal the thinking that led you to that point of view or to state the reasons why you think something is important.

To engage in a meaningful two-way conversation, it is important too to invite others to speak with their authentic voice, asking them to share how they see things and what leads them to see things in that way. As we shall discuss in the next chapter, assertiveness is the ability to state clearly and confidently what you want or need in a situation *and* to allow the other party to state clearly what he or she wants.

The first three conversational skills – listening, questioning and playing back – enable you to understand and explore the other person's position. The ability to voice your own views assertively enables you to set out your own position, and this is a vital skill in many contexts.

Difficult conversations

In *Difficult Conversations* Stone, Patton and Heen set out a framework to understand and to manage difficult conversations. A difficult conversation, they say, is anything you find it hard to talk about. For example, if someone finds it difficult to return a faulty item to a shop, then this is a difficult conversation, even though many other people might find this straightforward.

Stone, Patton and Heen's starting point is that any difficult conversation is actually three conversations:

- The 'What happened?' conversation: most difficult conversations involve disagreements about what has happened or what should happen.
- The feelings conversation: every difficult conversation also asks and answers questions about feelings. These feelings may not be addressed directly, but they will leak in anyway.

- **The identity conversation**: this is the conversation we each have with ourselves about what this situation means to us.

To illustrate these three conversations, imagine that you arranged to meet a friend for dinner in a local restaurant but she didn't show up and didn't contact you to let you know she wouldn't be there.

You speak to her the following day at the gym. She says that she thought this was just an idea that the two of you had spoken about without actually agreeing to meet. What might be going on for both of you during the conversation at the gym?

First, there is the 'What happened?' conversation. This might cover issues such as how clear it was that you'd agreed to meet, whether or not you should have confirmed arrangements, or what you might have done at the time when she didn't arrive.

Second, there is the 'feelings' conversation. This might never be articulated and one or both of you may not be conscious of your feelings. Nevertheless, there will be feelings present. For instance, you may feel disappointed or angry because you think she let you down. She may be upset because you seem to be attacking her without due cause. The nature of the relationship between you will influence how much these feelings are explored.

Third, there is the 'identity' conversation. This is probably even less likely to be voiced. Perhaps part of your identity is to see yourself as an honest, fair and reliable person who is also well organized. The conversation raised questions in your mind about how fair you're being and whether you are as well organized as you thought you were. Equally your friend sees herself as trustworthy and honest, and as a very supportive friend. This episode may cause her to question just how dependable she really is. Again the quality of the relationship between you will affect how far this conversation takes place. Even if nothing is said, each of you may be having part of this conversation in your own head.

Note the similarity between Stone, Patton and Heen's three conversations and the idea of listening with the head (for what happened), the heart (for feelings) and the gut (for questions of identity).

Tackling difficult conversations

Stone, Patton and Heen suggest that one way of engaging effectively in a difficult conversation is to move from a conversation about who is to blame to a conversation which is focused on learning for next time.

In a blame conversation, you are trying to prove that you were in the right and to place the blame largely or exclusively on the other person. This is likely to be met by some kind of resistance, and you probably end up in a conflict and a win–lose situation where even to 'win' might only be of short-term benefit.

Shifting to a mindset of engaging in a learning conversation means that your purpose changes and you want to share and understand different perspectives and look to construct positive ways forward that will benefit all parties. Shifting from message delivery to learning means that you stop arguing about who is right and start exploring each other's stories.

An important key to having a learning conversation is to distinguish blame from contribution. Rather than arguing about who is to blame, it is far more fruitful to explore what each of us contributed to the situation. Some of the differences in moving from blame to contribution are summarized below:

Who is to blame?	**What is my contribution?**
Seeks to judge others	Seeks to understand others
One-sided	Joint and interactive
Looks backwards	Looks forwards
Provokes defensiveness	Stimulates learning and change
Hinders problem-solving	Encourages problem-solving.

Stone, Patton and Heen write that:

> Talking about blame distracts us from exploring why things went wrong and how we might correct them going forward. Focusing instead on understanding the contribution system allows us to learn about the real causes of the problem, and to work on correcting them.

Exercise 5.3 From blame to contribution

Think of a conversation you had which became entrenched in both sides trying to blame or find fault in the other party.

- What was the outcome of the conversation?
- How did you feel at the end of it? How do you reckon the other person felt?
- What might you have said differently in order to explore the respective contributions of you and the other party?
- What would have been a useful attitude for you to adopt to create a contribution-type conversation?

Fierce conversations

In *Fierce Conversations* the American executive coach Susan Scott writes about conversations that get to the heart of the matter. By 'fierce' she does not mean aggressive but rather robust, passionate, eager.

Conversations that get to the heart of the matter, that surface assumptions and that explore different perspectives, take time. They might seem like an indulgence in today's fast-paced world where many people are very busy. However, the conversations that don't get to the heart of the matter in the end take up far more time because the decisions and actions 'agreed' in these conversations don't address the full reality of the situation. Susan Scott writes that 'fierce conversations often do take time. The problem is, anything else takes longer.'

I sometimes share with a coaching client the following exercise from Susan Scott's book. I ask my client to think of a difficult conversation he or she would like to have. I then invite my client to prepare an opening statement lasting just 60 seconds covering these seven elements:

1 Name the issue.
2 Select a specific example that illustrates the behaviour or situation you want to change.
3 Describe your emotions about the issue.

4 Clarify what is at stake.
5 Identify your contribution to this problem.
6 Indicate your wish to resolve the issue.
7 Invite your partner to respond.

Susan Scott argues that it is possible to cover all of these points in 60 seconds as a way of setting up a fierce or difficult conversation. Here is an illustration of the seven steps in a scenario where a parent is confronting her teenage son about coming home late:

> I'd like to speak to you about your not coming home till after midnight. [1] On Friday I heard you open the front door after 2 a.m. [2] I'm disappointed that you're breaking our rule that you have to be home by midnight, and I also become very anxious when you're out so late and I haven't heard from you. [3] The exam season is about to start and it's important that you're feeling refreshed so that you can revise. [4] I realize that I haven't brought this up before now even though this has been going on for several months. [5] I want us to agree what time you will be home when you're out with friends, and what you will do to let me know that you're going to be late. [6] Now I'd like to hear what you think. [7]

I find that the idea of saying all of this in one minute without being interrupted strikes many people as a bit unrealistic. However, noting what they'd like to say under each heading is very useful in helping them to clarify the key points they'd like to cover in the conversation.

I then invite the client to rehearse this opening statement, and together we review how assertively he or she was able to make this. I may offer some feedback on what came across to me as powerful or weak, or on things like tone of voice or hesitancy of speech. The client then makes the statement a second time, incorporating the points taken from the review.

Note that the above seven steps only set up the conversation. To actually have the conversation in reality, you also need to:

1 interact with the other person, and in particular find out his or her views;
2 seek to jointly resolve the issue, emphasizing how you can both move forward;
3 reach an agreement.

Exercise 5.4 Preparing for a fierce conversation

Think of a situation – ideally a current one, though you could consider something from the past if you wish – where it would be useful to have an honest but difficult conversation with someone. Make some notes to prepare a one-minute introduction setting up the conversation:

1 Name the issue.
2 Select a specific example that illustrates the behaviour or situation you want to change.
3 Describe your emotions about the issue.
4 Clarify what is at stake.
5 Identify your contribution to this problem.
6 Indicate your wish to resolve the issue.
7 Invite your partner to respond.

If you do have the conversation, you might not go through all seven steps in one minute. Nevertheless, the exercise will help to clarify the key points you want to raise in the conversation.

6

Assertiveness and handling conflict

Introduction

In this chapter we shall look at two topics in which the ability to be aware of and to manage what is going on within yourself is deeply connected to your ability to interact successfully with other people. We begin with assertiveness, and consider the difference between assertive, aggressive and passive behaviour. This links closely to your ability to manage conflict, and we shall explore five different ways in which you might handle conflict. These are two areas where many people struggle and hence are topics that are often raised in coaching sessions.

People who find it difficult to be assertive frequently find it hard to say no to any request. Hence they take on too much, which may cause them problems with time management, finding a desirable work–life balance, or stress. One of the classic books on assertiveness, written by Manuel Smith, has the title *When I Say No I Feel Guilty*. This suggests that problems in being assertive may have their roots deep in someone's early experiences and personality. However, we won't be looking at these ideas in a psychodynamic or therapeutic way. Rather, as with the other ideas explored in the book, we introduce the notion of assertiveness to invite you, first, to think about your situation with a fresh eye and then, if you choose, to behave in new ways. In other words, we hope that the ideas explored below will raise your awareness and encourage you to take responsibility for doing things differently.

Assertive, aggressive and passive behaviour

In everyday language when people describe someone as 'assertive' they often mean that this person is good at getting his or her own way. I shall use the word 'aggressive' rather than 'assertive' to describe such behaviour.

Here is a definition of **assertiveness** that we shall use throughout this chapter:

> Assertiveness is the ability to state clearly and confidently what you want or need in a situation *and* to allow the other party to state clearly what he or she wants.

Thus behaving assertively is about equality and mutuality rather than simply getting your own way.

Behaving **passively** means that you are unable to ask for what you want or to insist upon getting what you are entitled to. Over the years I have run many workshops on assertiveness. I cannot recall a single instance of someone coming on the workshop because they felt their behaviour was too aggressive. It's passive people who come to assertiveness workshops.

Figure 6.1 illustrates the distinction between assertive, aggressive and passive behaviour.

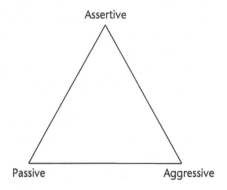

Assertive

Passive   Aggressive

Figure 6.1 Assertive, aggressive and passive

There are occasions when it is wise to be passive – for example, if you are faced with overwhelming odds. And there are times when it is important to be aggressive and fight for what you want – for instance, insisting that a doctor pays a home visit to your very sick child. However, in most situations behaving assertively is a useful and healthy thing to do.

It is often the case that someone who behaves passively is, in Transactional Analysis terms, operating from an Adapted Child ego state. Consciously striving to remain in Adult, inviting the other person to respond from his or her Adult ego state, can help that person to behave more assertively.

Basic assertiveness

An alternative term for what we've called 'aggressiveness' is 'basic assertiveness'. **Basic assertiveness** might be defined as the first half of the above definition – the ability to state clearly and confidently what you want or need in a situation. When you behave with basic assertiveness, you do not take into account the needs of the other party. As an illustration, you might take a basic assertive stance when returning a faulty item to a shop. Hopefully you treat the shop assistant courteously, but you are not concerned about the relationship between you, which is a very temporary one, nor with the assistant's needs.

If, however, you are dealing with a friend, relative, neighbour, work colleague or client, then the health of the relationship between the two of you may be important, and it is extremely useful if you can behave with genuine assertiveness in your interactions with the other person.

I find it useful to think of assertiveness as a two-way street whereas aggressiveness or basic assertiveness is a one-way street.

If you find it difficult to be assertive, then it is possible to learn to become more so. One technique which can be helpful when you wish to be basically assertive is known as the **broken record**. The metaphor comes from the time when recorded music was played back on black vinyl records. Sometimes, if the record was slightly damaged, the needle on the record player would become stuck and the same small piece of the song would be played back repeatedly. When you use the broken record technique you simply repeat the same phrase in response to whatever objection the other party makes. As an example, if you are returning a faulty item to a shop, repeatedly stating 'This item is faulty and I want my money back' can be very hard for the other person to resist.

Rights and responsibilities

A useful idea in assertiveness is the notion of **rights**. As a human being, you have rights, such as the right to:

- state your opinion;
- get what you pay for;
- ask for what you want;
- say no;
- change your mind;
- make a mistake;
- be treated with respect;
- choose not to assert yourself.

Even though you may have less authority and power than, for example, the head teacher of your children's school or the chief executive of the organization where you work, nevertheless you are their equal simply because each of you is a human being.

Exercise 6.1 Your rights

Which of these rights do you find it difficult to permit yourself?

- State your opinion.
- Get what you pay for.
- Ask for what you want.
- Say no.
- Change your mind.
- Make a mistake.
- Be treated with respect.
- Choose not to assert yourself.

What other rights do you not allow yourself?

Alongside these rights you also have **responsibilities**, and you have to live with the consequences of your actions. For example, when your manager asks you to work overtime you might say no because you have an important private engagement that evening. However, if you regularly say no to reasonable requests from your boss, then you may find yourself having to look for a new job. Similarly, if you frequently break arrangements to meet friends, then you will soon acquire a reputation for being unreliable.

Developing assertive behaviours

One way in which I sometimes work with coaching clients who are having difficulties in being assertive is to invite them to rehearse with me a conversation they would like to have with someone but which they are putting off. The person prepares and then delivers her assertive statement, and together we review how she performed. I usually ask the person to give herself feedback before adding any comments of my own. Then the client has another attempt, building in her learning from the review.

One thing which often emerges in such a rehearsal is the importance of body language and tone of voice in speaking assertively. Assertive people take space – literally and metaphorically – to deliver their message. If you watch someone like Barack Obama giving a speech you will notice that he actually speaks very slowly, taking lots of time and space to give his message. It is important to take your time to speak in a confident, clear voice.

There are two things which often make a statement more assertive. The first is to explain the reasons behind your views or to state why something is important to you. The second – which may not be appropriate in some settings – is to state how you feel about a situation. To illustrate these points, compare these statements:

- I won't be able to help at the school fete.
- I won't be able to help at the school fete because I'm going to my niece's wedding.

- I can't talk to you now.
- I can't talk to you now because I'm very upset.

Another point which is very helpful in speaking assertively is to make sure that you don't dilute your message. I frequently find that people rehearsing a statement start with a clear expression of

their views and then go on to add lots of detail, explanation or jus-
tification. Indeed, they may in effect talk themselves out of what
they initially asked for. It is really useful to make a simple, crisp
statement, setting out your view or asking simply and directly for
what you want.

Here is a summary of some of the tips set out above:

- Ask simply and directly for what you wish for.
- Don't dilute your message with long explanations or just-
  ifications.
- Avoid unnecessary apologies or putting yourself down.
- Notice your body language – take your time to speak in a confi-
  dent, clear voice.
- Don't allow others to make unreasonable demands on you.
- Say no without feeling guilty.

When you have behaved passively for many years, beginning to
behave more assertively can seem to you to be aggressive. It can
also surprise other people around you who may have benefited
from your lack of assertiveness in the past.

Exercise 6.2 Behaving more assertively

Think of a situation where you find it difficult to behave assertively.

- Which of the ideas mentioned above might help you?
- What specifically will you try out in order to be more assertive?

You will find it useful to reflect upon and learn from what happens when
you try these ideas out. Learning to behave assertively may involve breaking habits that are well established. I encourage you not to be over-critical
of your performance but rather to persevere in experimenting with your
new behaviours.

Handling conflict

We turn now to consider how passive, aggressive and assertive
behaviour relates to different ways of handling conflict.

I find the following short definition very useful:

Conflict is any form of disagreement, no matter how large or small.

As Figure 6.2 indicates, conflict which isn't addressed can escalate over time. What starts as mild irritation may become annoyance, perhaps leading to anger and possibly violence. Hence, it is easier to tackle conflict in its early stages. However, most people prefer to settle for an easier life, say nothing and hope that the disagreement will go away or resolve itself. This does sometimes happen, but the risk in not addressing problems is that they get worse and so become more difficult to solve.

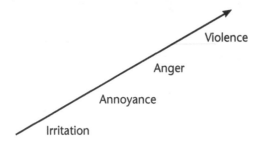

Figure 6.2 Conflict may escalate

When people describe their situation as a disagreement or conflict with a colleague or manager, I am likely to draw the diagram in Figure 6.3 which shows five possible styles of handling conflict. This was originally described by two writers, Kenneth Thomas and Ralph Kilmann, and the framework is known as the Thomas–Kilmann model. I think it is a really useful framework to help you think about how you handle conflict and how you might behave differently and more effectively.

The five styles depend on whether you attempt to satisfy the needs of yourself or the needs of the other party.

- If you seek to satisfy your own needs and disregard the needs of the other party, then the style is described as **competing**.
- However, if you give priority to satisfying the needs of the other person and disregard your own needs, then this is described as **accommodating**.

- If you make no attempt to satisfy either your own or the other party's needs, then this is referred to as **avoiding**.
- On the other hand, if you endeavour to meet both your own needs and the needs of the other person, this is called **collaborating**.
- Finally, if you seek to meet some of your needs and some of the other party's – splitting the difference in some way, as it were – then this is called **compromising**.

Needs of others

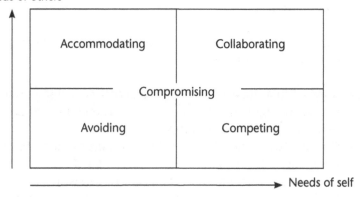

Figure 6.3 **Five ways of handling conflict**

The different styles of handling conflict are related to the idea of passive, assertive and aggressive behaviours that we looked at earlier in the chapter. Behaving passively means that you don't attempt to meet your needs, which equates to avoiding or accommodating. Aggressive behaviour – or what we called basic assertiveness – is similar to competing to get what you want. And being genuinely assertive is required in seeking a collaborative outcome where you and the other party are both satisfied.

The styles are also linked to notions of winning and losing. Collaboration is a search for a win–win outcome. In avoiding, we both lose as the situation is not resolved. Competing can be viewed as win–lose, while accommodating is lose–win.

Let me illustrate the five styles with a simple example where there is an orange available to you and me.

- If we are both too embarrassed to say we would like the orange, then neither of us gets it and we are avoiding.
- If I simply hand over the orange to you, I am accommodating.
- If I arm-wrestle with you to win the orange for myself, I am competing.
- If we cut the orange in two (not necessarily equal) parts and share it, we are compromising.
- If we explore why each of us wants the orange and realize that you need only the flesh for juice while I need only the peel for a cookery recipe, then we can both get what we want and we are collaborating.

It is important to note that each of these styles can be appropriate depending on the situation.

- If we are in a situation where the outcome is very important to you but not particularly important to me, then I might usefully decide to accommodate your wishes.
- On the other hand, if it is really important to me to have my needs met – for instance, I may have applied for a job that I really want – then I need to compete to try to win.
- If I have absolutely no chance of getting what I want, then it would be wise to avoid the conflict. Or, if there is no chance of reaching agreement today but a good chance of agreeing next time we meet, then I might avoid the issue for the time being.
- Some situations lend themselves naturally to compromise. Negotiations – for instance, between management and trade unions – often go through a somewhat ritualistic offer and counter-offer before a compromise is reached. Management offers a 2 per cent pay rise, the trade union demands 10 per cent, and a settlement of 4 per cent is reached in due course. Or imagine that you put your house on the market for £300,000, receive an offer of £270,000, and eventually agree to sell the house for £290,000.
- There are times when it may be very important to seek a collaborative outcome. For example, if you and I hope to establish a long-term business or personal partnership, then it may be vital that we explore in depth what each of us seeks from the

arrangement and only agree when we both feel satisfied that our needs are being well served. Note that it often isn't possible to reach a collaborative agreement – wage bargaining might well be one such situation.

The person who is best equipped to handle conflict well is one who can use all of the styles effectively and who knows which style is most appropriate in any situation. It's a bit like having a number of golf clubs in your bag – the really good player knows when to select each of the clubs, and can use all of them skilfully.

Exercise 6.3 Appreciating another point of view

We have defined conflict as any form of disagreement, however large or small. Think of a current situation in which your wishes differ from those of others. Or take a recent situation in which you were in conflict with another individual or group of people. Make some notes in answer to these questions:

- What is the situation?
- Who is involved?
- What do you really want?
- What are your concerns?
- What do you think the other person really wants?
- What are that person's concerns?
- What can you do to check out his or her position?
- What, if anything, will you do to address the conflict between you?

In the previous chapter on conversations, we looked at how you might have a difficult conversation with someone. The ideas explored there are useful when tackling a conflict situation too.

Principled negotiation

One approach to seeking a collaborative, win–win outcome is the idea of principled negotiation. This was set out in a classic book by Roger Fisher and William Ury called *Getting to Yes*. Fisher and Ury set out four fundamental principles of principled negotiation:

1 Separate the people from the problem – deal with relationship issues separately from the substantive issues.
2 Focus on interests, not positions – negotiate about things that people really want and need, not what they say they want or need.
3 Invent options for mutual gain – look to create solutions that allow both sides to win.
4 Insist on objective criteria – if possible, establish some objective criteria to assess whether an agreement is fair.

Let's look at their second point, focusing on interests rather than negotiating from entrenched positions. When you negotiate about interests, you seek to establish what you and the other party really want, not what she initially says she wants. Exploring what really matters to both parties may reveal that the underlying interests and needs of both parties are actually compatible, not mutually exclusive.

To engage in principled negotiation is to take part in a dialogue rather than a debate. Debate assumes that there is a single right answer – generally one's own – and that the goal is to find this answer or to win the argument. Debate is about winning or losing, or perhaps compromising.

In contrast, dialogue assumes that there are multiple perspectives, and the goal is to explore these different viewpoints in order to understand each other's position. It is about exploring ideas together, generating fresh insights and creating new possibilities. Dialogue is about searching creatively for win–win outcomes.

Participants in a dialogue are curious about each other's views, looking for what's new or what they can learn. They listen in order to understand, they ask open questions to deepen their understanding, and they play back what they've heard to the other party. They are also able to voice their own position assertively. By sharing perspectives and surfacing assumptions they begin to create new possibilities that respect the views and needs of everyone involved. These are the four skills of listening, questioning, playing back and voicing that we explored in the previous chapter on conversations.

7

Influencing

To operate effectively you often need to obtain the consent of, or buy in from, people over whom you do not have authority. In this chapter we shall consider how you might use different styles and approaches in order to influence other people or to gain their genuine commitment.

Influencing may be defined as the ability to affect attitude, behaviour or outcomes. To illustrate the difference between these three aspects, you might imagine a teacher seeking to help a pupil feel more positive about staying on at school (attitude) or to encourage him to spend more time on homework (behaviour) or to help him to achieve better exam grades (outcome). Clearly each of the three aspects is to some extent dependent on the other two.

Some people are very good at presenting a logical case with a reasoned statement of costs and benefits. In some situations this is effective, but someone who can only work with logic will be limited in his or her ability to influence others. As with many other aspects of interpersonal behaviour – such as handling conflict, which we considered in the previous chapter – it is very useful to have a range of styles, together with the ability to choose flexibly one that is appropriate to the situation.

Influencing tactics

Here is a simple model showing seven possible tactics you could use to influence someone.

- Reason – logical presentation of ideas.
- Friendliness – creation of goodwill.
- Coalition – getting the support of others to back up requests.
- Bargaining – negotiating or trading.
- Forcefulness – a direct approach, ordering and demanding

compliance. This is akin to basic assertiveness.

- Higher authority – getting the support of individuals higher up in the hierarchy or pecking order.
- Sanctions – use of rewards and punishments, carrots and sticks. Some of these might be intangible, such as praise or criticism.

Exercise 7.1 invites you to consider which of these tactics you employ and which tactics you could usefully deploy more often.

Exercise 7.1 What tactics do you use to influence people?

Which of the seven tactics do you employ frequently, sometimes, occasionally or never?

Table 7.1 How often do you use these tactics?

Tactic	Never, occasionally, sometimes or often?
Reason – logical presentation of ideas	
Friendliness – creation of goodwill	
Coalition – getting the support of others to back up requests	
Bargaining – negotiating	
Assertiveness – a direct approach, ordering and demanding compliance	
Higher authority – getting the support of individuals higher up	
Sanctions – use of rewards and punishments	

Which tactics will you use more than you do at present?

Four approaches to influencing

Roger Harrison and David Berlew developed a more detailed framework based on four different approaches to influencing.

- Assertive persuasion
- Reward and punishment
- Participation and trust
- Common vision.

Note that the word 'assertive' here is being used in the sense of basic assertiveness rather than the mutual, two-way notion of assertiveness that we looked at in the previous chapter. Let's consider the four approaches in turn.

Assertive persuasion

This is the most common approach to influencing in meetings, and is akin to the use of logical argument. It consists of presenting ideas or suggestions, and giving the reasons or facts which support this view. It also involves putting forward arguments or facts to counter opposing views. In terms of the ladder of listening that we looked at in Chapter 5, it involves listening to disagree rather than listening to understand. It may involve asking leading questions rather than open questions.

Reward and punishment

This approach involves the use of some combination of sticks and carrots to shape the behaviour of others. As an illustration, you might offer to pay some money to your teenage son or daughter to do some gardening for you, or you might ground them for a week for misbehaving. In a work context, the threat of losing your job is a powerful illustration of the stick variety, while bonus schemes or promises of promotion are incentives of the carrot variety. The use of reward and punishment can also be the basis of bargaining between parties.

It is, of course, necessary to be in a position where you can offer such sticks and carrots. They may be common practice in some organizations – one thinks of bankers' bonuses – but less common in others. Moreover, the effectiveness of the approach depends on how much importance the other party attaches to the incentives.

Rewards and punishments can be psychological as well as tangible – for instance, giving praise or showing respect, on the one hand, or criticism or rejection, on the other. The use of reward and punishment can at times produce an unhealthy climate of threat and competition within an organization.

Participation and trust

This is a softer style of influencing which seeks to win the commitment of others and establish a collaborative style of working. It might be used when there is no possibility of demanding compliance or of using rewards and punishment. It might also be particularly appropriate when it is vital to win genuine commitment.

Establishing an atmosphere of trust is likely to require giving up close control of the work of the other party. Rather, the influencer seeks other people's ideas and is willing to share responsibility with them. This approach involves listening to understand what is most important to the other, and playing back this understanding.

Common vision

This approach seeks to focus the energies of a group on a common goal, which in some situations might be to win against a rival group. Winston Churchill's leadership of the British people in the Second World War is a vivid example of this.

The approach is potentially very powerful but is effective in a more limited range of situations than the other styles. It seeks to draw on the values, emotions and aspirations of the group. This is more likely to be successful when the influencer is perceived genuinely to share these interests. It is unlikely to work if the influencer does not have the trust of the group.

To generate a compelling vision requires an enthusiastic painting of future possibilities which generates excitement, commitment and connection in others.

Exercise 7.2 Choosing an approach to influencing

Identify a situation where you wish to influence the behaviour of others or the outcome of a project. Make notes in answer to these questions:

- What is the result you want?
- Whom do you need to influence to achieve this result?
- Which of the four approaches will you adopt?
- What specifically will you do to achieve the result you are looking for?

Authority, presence and impact

In *Coaching, Mentoring and Organizational Consultancy* Peter Hawkins and Nick Smith suggest that there are three aspects of personal power and influence – authority, presence and impact (see Figure 7.1).

- Your **authority** is based on your achievements. It is about what you have done in the past.
- Your **presence** is based on your ability to command respect and attention. It is about how you are now.
- Your **impact** is based on what you are able to make happen. It is about what you will change in the future.

Hawkins and Smith write that:

> Authority is about our credibility. It can derive from what, or who, you know or what you have done in the past . . .
>
> Presence involves creating relationship and community. It is the ability to be fully present with a quality of immediacy and to develop relationship and rapport quickly and with very different types of people . . .
>
> People with high levels of impact can shift the direction of a meeting, conversation or event. They have the ability to intervene in a way that shifts or reframes the way issues under discussion are being perceived and addressed.

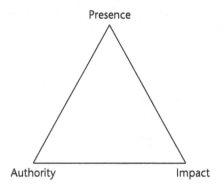

Figure 7.1 Authority, presence and impact

As an oversimplified illustration – based on public perception only, it must be said – of these aspects, consider three British prime ministers. When he took over the premiership Gordon Brown had authority based on his earlier achievements as Chancellor of the Exchequer. Tony Blair had presence, with the ability to command the attention of everyone in a room. Margaret Thatcher had impact – she changed things, for instance through her privatization programme. Note that I'm not making any political points whatsoever here about the desirability or otherwise of what each of them did.

And Nelson Mandela had all three – authority, presence and impact!

I think that authority, presence and impact are relative terms. For example, I once heard a former leader of the Conservative Party speak without notes for an hour, commanding the attention of 500 people. Yet he didn't come across to the general British public as a credible contender for prime minister when he was leader of the Opposition. It is often the case that people who can command attention at one level in an organization or community aren't able to do so at a higher level of leadership.

Stakeholder analysis

A useful exercise when you embark on a project where you will need to influence others is to identify and then analyse the various stakeholders involved. A stakeholder is anyone who has a vested interest in your project or who will be affected by its outcomes. Stakeholders may be within or external to your organization.

There are various ways in which you might characterize the stakeholders and map them on to a grid such as the one shown in Figure 7.2. This distinguishes those stakeholders who have high or low power over the decision to proceed or over the success of your project, and those who have high or low interest in your project.

You need to tailor your communications and interactions differently to each group. For example:

- **High power, interested** people: these are the people you must fully engage with and make the greatest efforts to satisfy. You may wish to actively involve these people in your plans.
- **High power, less interested** people: you need to put in enough work with these people to keep them satisfied, but not so much that they become bored with your message. You will need to address any concerns they may have.
- **Low power, interested** people: keep these people adequately informed, and talk to them to ensure that no major issues are arising. These people can often be very helpful with the detail of your project.
- **Low power, less interested** people: again, monitor these people, but do not bore them with excessive communication.

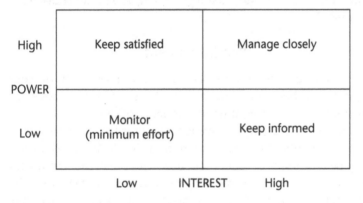

Figure 7.2 Stakeholder mapping

Note too that it is important to think about your stakeholders as the project develops, not just at the start. It can help from time to time to revisit your analysis, and consider the extent to which you have the key stakeholders on board and what else you need to do to communicate with or involve them.

Exercise 7.3 Stakeholder analysis

Identify a project that you are working on or a piece of work that is important to you.

1 List the key stakeholders – that is, the people who have an interest in your project or who will be affected by it.
2 Put yourself in the shoes of each stakeholder in turn. What are the pros and cons of your project from his or her perspective?
3 On a scale of 1 (low) to 10 (high), rank each stakeholder in terms of his or her:
   – interest – that is, how much each one cares about your project;
   – power – that is, each one's ability to affect the success of your project.
4 What will you do to manage each of the high-interest, high-power stakeholders?
5 What will you do to keep the low-interest, high-power stakeholders satisfied?
6 What will you do to keep the high-interest, low-power stakeholders informed?

Self-assessment

This section invites you to do one more assessment of your approach to influencing. The table in Exercise 7.4 describes eight behaviours that you might use to influence others.

There are three aspects of influencing reflected in these behavioural statements. The first is the notion that to influence others it may be important to build their views and preferences into your proposals. To influence someone you need to start from where he or she is. People do things for reasons that they think are sensible, and their reasoning may be different from yours. And people take in information that makes sense to them, which may differ from the information which you think is important.

The second element is the idea that you have to be flexible in your approach. We looked earlier in the chapter at different tactics and approaches that you might use.

The final aspect within the statements is that it is very helpful to present your views clearly and confidently. Gravitas is a tricky concept to pin down. You often know it when you see it, and you may be aware that it's lacking without necessarily being able to define what's missing.

You might like to consider how well you influence others by assessing yourself against the statements in Exercise 7.4. You could also gather feedback from others by asking them to rate you against the eight statements in Table 7.2.

Exercise 7.4 Assessment of influencing skills

To assess your influencing skills, indicate your agreement or disagreement with each of the statements in Table 7.2, using this five-point scale:

1 Strongly disagree.
2 Disagree.
3 Neither agree nor disagree.
4 Agree.
5 Strongly agree.

Reflecting on your own ratings – and the ratings of others if you have gathered feedback – what will you do differently to influence others more effectively?

Table 7.2 How influential are you?

I consciously involve and consult key players at an early stage and build their preferences into decisions.

I take pains to build consensus with key stakeholders around the best way forward.

I create highly effective relationships with a wide range of people, particularly those in senior positions.

I use a variety of approaches, and work convincingly with both logic and emotion to persuade and influence others.

I generally judge effectively when to persist and when to give way.

I impress others, particularly senior people, as someone with gravitas and sound judgement.

I say clearly, assertively and succinctly what I mean or what I want.

I present a compelling case in both one-to-one and group situations, even when there is opposition to my views.

Managing upwards

When I ran workshops on coaching skills for managers in the gas pipeline company Transco, a question that was often asked by one of the participants was 'How do I coach my boss?' Invariably, with a little probing it became clear that what the participant really wanted was to get the boss in question to do what that individual wanted. As we considered in Chapter 1, coaching is about helping the other person to clarify his or her goals and work out how to achieve them. These participants didn't want to coach their bosses – they wanted to influence them.

Managing your boss, or more generally managing upwards within your organization, is one important aspect of influencing. The ideas explored earlier in the chapter apply here too. To influence your boss, you need to appreciate the world from his or her perspective, and you need to work out – perhaps through experience of what does and doesn't work – what styles or tactics are effective in persuading your boss to buy into your ideas.

There is one other point that is very important in managing your boss. You need to be delivering successfully on the objectives that your manager has asked you to work on. If you have a reputation with your boss as a reliable member of her team, then it will be much easier to sell your ideas to her. If, on the other hand, your manager reckons that you don't deliver, then it will be very difficult to influence her. The foundation for managing upwards is to build yourself a reputation for good performance.

8

Managing your time

Introduction

Many years ago, before I became involved in management development, I attended a two-day time management course. It was a well-run programme, and I found it useful. For me, the mark of a successful course is that you as a participant gain one thing that you are still using years later. I'll tell you shortly what I took from that course. However, even as the course was unfolding I realized that we were looking at time management at two levels. At some points we were considering things philosophically as we explored what really mattered to each of us and how this was reflected in how we spent our time. At other points on the course the facilitator was introducing us to various tips on time management and how to use a personal organizer effectively. This was in the days when Filofaxes, etc., were relatively new.

In this chapter I want to look at time management mainly from the first of these points of view. I remember leaving the course with a brand new Filofax and all the tailored pieces of paper to populate it. I do know people who find this type of personal organizer very useful. However, I personally never took mine out of the box and so never learnt whether or not it would work for me.

The thing which I myself took from the course and which I still practise, literally decades later, is that the key to managing your time effectively is to know your priorities and then spend your time in ways which reflect those priorities. It is as simple, as profound and as difficult as that! When I run workshops on time management or when I work with coaching clients on how they manage their time, that is the fundamental idea I am offering. In this chapter I'll invite you to clarify for yourself what activities are most important to you.

Your priorities

Since I regard this as the key to managing your time effectively, let me say it again in slightly different words. There are two basic things you need to do to manage your time:

- First, be clear about what your priorities are.
- Second, spend your time in ways which reflect your priorities.

This raises the question of who sets your priorities. I realize – not least because I am in this position myself – that you may be working within an organization and hence required to deliver objectives on behalf of the organization or set by your boss. Or you may be juggling the demands of bringing up a family, running a household and looking after elderly relatives. And you have bills and maybe a mortgage to pay each month. There are real constraints on your freedom to choose your priorities. Your view on your priorities must reflect these constraints and perhaps the needs of some other people. Nevertheless, I suggest that ultimately you choose your priorities. It is your choice to stay in that organization or to live in that house, for instance. I don't want to come across as naïve here. I do recognize that at the time of writing – in the midst of the worst recession in living memory – it isn't easy to change jobs or even move house. But I suggest that ultimately you are the decision-maker about what your priorities are. *It's your life!*

This extends in particular to how you balance your time between work and non-work activities – if you are in work, that is. Given the constraints imposed by your job or of running your own business, together with time spent travelling to work, how do you want to split your time between working and doing other things?

In terms of priorities in general, and work–life balance in particular, my own view is that there are no right answers – there are only your answers. Some individuals thrive on a 14-hour working day. For them it may be that, in the words of Noël Coward, 'Work is more fun than fun.' For many people, the thought of a 14-hour working day would be a nightmare. But it's a personal choice how much time you'd like to spend working. And if you are working a 14-hour day and hating it, then you might want to consider making some changes. So let's look now at an idea which might help if, like many people today, you're seeking a work–life balance which has less work and more life in it.

Urgent versus important

Stephen Covey's best selling book *The 7 Habits of Highly Effective People* describes seven habits to help people live balanced and fulfilled lives. The first three habits are concerned with personal effectiveness, the next three with interpersonal relationships, and the final one is about constantly renewing the other habits. His seven habits are:

1 **Be proactive.** Take responsibility for your life and your choices. Show initiative. Don't blame others or circumstances.
2 **Begin with the end in mind.** What do you want to be remembered for? What do you really, really want?
3 **Put first things first.** Identify and follow your priorities. This is the key to time management.
4 **Think win–win.** Look for agreements or solutions that are mutually beneficial. Seek to collaborate rather than compete.
5 **Seek first to understand, then to be understood.** Take time to listen to understand the other person's perceptions and priorities. Listen for feelings and meanings, not just facts and logic. Then express your own views clearly.
6 **Synergy.** Creative cooperation means that 1 + 1 can equal 3 or more. Honest communication and a valuing of differences mean that new possibilities can be created.
7 **Renewal.** Maintenance is essential. Keep the habits alive by continually attending to them, and by continually developing and renewing yourself.

Let's look in more detail at Covey's third habit: put first things first. He introduces the distinction between activities which are urgent and activities which are important. This leads to the 2 × 2 matrix shown in Figure 8.1.

Most people are good at attending to activities which are both urgent and important. Crises, deadlines and important meetings are examples of things which generally are dealt with. What really distinguishes people who are good at managing their time is that they also focus on things which are important but not yet urgent. Most of the rest of us focus on activities which are urgent but not necessarily important – interruptions, meetings where we don't really need to be present, some phone calls, many emails, and so on. And, if you are spending much time on things which are neither urgent nor important, then you're not using your time very wisely at all.

It is interesting to note the activities which Covey puts in the 'important but not urgent' box. Many of these activities, such as preparation, planning and empowering others, might be regarded as investments of time – that is, time spent now which will yield dividends later. He also adds the term 're-creation' – that is, the activities you do to re-create yourself. These are the things you do to relax and recharge your batteries, which will vary from person to person. He's suggesting, for instance, that a ten-minute walk in the fresh air might be a really good use of your time if it helps you to be more productive later. And he considers building relationships an important activity that generally isn't urgent. For example, it

	Urgent	Not urgent
Important	Crises Pressing problems Deadline-driven projects Some meetings	Preparation Prevention Planning Relationship building Re-creation Empowerment
Not important	Interruptions Some phone calls Some mail or reports Some meetings Some 'pressing matters' Many popular activities	Trivia, busywork Junk mail Some phone calls Time wasters 'Escape' activities

Figure 8.1 Urgent versus important

may not matter if you don't have coffee with a new colleague or neighbour this week – it isn't urgent. But if you continually postpone this, then you may have missed an opportunity to develop a relationship that may be of great benefit at some point in the future.

I sometimes invite a coaching client to make a list of the activities which make up his or her working week and then to put them into these four boxes. I regard the client as the judge of what is and isn't important. It is common to find that people view most of the things that they do as important. However, importance is a relative concept – some things are more important than others, and everything can't be top priority, by definition. Even bearing this in mind, however, people are reluctant to relegate activities to 'not that important'. However, if you want to manage your time effectively and strategically, then you need to clarify what you really do see as important. And you need to invest time in those things which are important but not yet urgent. One consequence of this is that fewer things will end up in the 'important and urgent' box since you've dealt with them well before the deadline.

Exercise 8.1 What's important to you?

What are the most important things that you do? And what are the things that are important to you but which you don't actually now do?

- List these things in descending order of how important they are to you.
- In a typical week, how much time do you spend on these important things?
- Now list these things again in descending order of how much time you spend on them.

Comparing the two lists, identify those areas where you would like to spend more time and where you would like to spend less time.

Exercise 8.2 on p. 80 is designed to give you a more accurate estimate of how much time you spend on different activities.

Schedule your priorities

One way of shifting how you spend your time so that you focus on the important rather than the urgent can be summed up in the phrase: 'Schedule your priorities, don't prioritize your schedule.' Just because a meeting is in your diary or a task is on your 'to do' list, that doesn't necessarily mean that it is important. But many people run from one meeting to another somewhat unthinkingly because it's in their calendar. I suggest you question the notion that you have to prioritize what's in your schedule.

On the other hand, putting things into your diary which are important but not urgent increases the likelihood that you will indeed invest time in these activities. A common example of this is the writing of an important report. Most people need a decent amount of fairly uninterrupted time to write significant pieces. This can be difficult to do if your day is full of meetings, phone calls, emails and colleagues or friends dropping by. It can be very effective to set aside a block of time and to find a suitable venue – possibly working from home if that's feasible – to do this kind of writing.

Another example is booking a meeting with yourself in your calendar. This might be time for planning or preparation or simply thinking time. Treat this meeting as you would any other important meeting. For instance, have a start and finish time, expect not to be interrupted for matters that aren't serious, don't take phone calls or deal with emails during the meeting, and only cancel – or postpone – the meeting for something else that's important.

I still recall an analogy offered by the facilitator on the time management workshop I attended all those years ago. To illustrate the notion of scheduling your priorities, imagine that you are about to pack the boot of your car to go on holiday. (If you don't drive, you can still imagine that a friend has offered to drive you to your destination.) Let's say you have two large suitcases containing the things you will really need on holiday and a dozen carrier bags with things that are nice to have – maybe a pair of spare flip-flops, a set of boules you occasionally play with, a disposable barbecue, and so on. How do you pack the boot? If you put all the carrier bags in first, you might well find that there's room for only one of the suitcases – some of the important stuff won't get in. Alternatively, you can pack the two suitcases first and then see how many of the carriers bags can be fitted in. It doesn't really matter if one or two carrier bags have to be left behind. Similarly, in scheduling your priorities and in working through your 'to do' list, make sure you devote sufficiently large chunks of time to carrying out the large, important tasks. Then fit the less important tasks around the larger, scheduled priorities. As an illustration, you might have five minutes to spare when you can fit in a phone call or deal with a number of emails.

Note that it isn't enough just to schedule your priorities. You also have to make sure you carry out the priority activities that you have scheduled. Having good intentions is a useful first step, but isn't enough.

A word that I like to use when talking about time management is 'ruthless'. I think it's helpful to be ruthless when prioritizing and when scheduling your priorities. By ruthless, I don't mean cruel or unfeeling. Rather, I mean having a very clear focus and determination. If you have lots of demands on your time, it is even more important to focus very clearly on what you regard as the really worthwhile uses of your time.

One of the skills which will help you in scheduling your priorities is the ability to say no. This is not about ignoring the needs of other people, and can be consistent with Covey's fourth habit of seeking win–win outcomes. Rather, it is about being assertive. Recall that in Chapter 6 on assertiveness we put forward this definition:

Assertiveness is the ability to state clearly and confidently what you want or need in a situation *and* to allow the other party to state clearly what he or she wants.

If you want to manage your time effectively and strategically, achieving the work–life balance that you seek, then it is important to be able assertively to say no to requests or activities that you judge to be relatively less important. I realize that it can be difficult to say no without feeling guilty – or that you're letting others down. I also recognize that there are occasions when it is unwise or hurtful to say no, and you may choose to go along with a request that you'd rather decline. Nevertheless, the ability at times to say no can be invaluable in focusing your efforts on the things that really matter.

I mentioned above that I myself never started to use the Filofax given out on the time management course. I do, however, believe that it's very helpful to have some kind of system to organize your time and your tasks. For some people, this kind of personal organizer works well. I encourage you to develop a system that suits you personally. I myself use a calendar on my PC to keep my diary, a spreadsheet to keep contact details, and a sheet of A4 paper to capture the tasks on my 'to do' list. Not very sophisticated, but it works for me.

A time log exercise

An activity that you might like to carry out is to complete a log of how you spend your time over a fairly typical week. Create a blank table with seven columns representing seven days and with as many rows as you need to split your wakeful time into half-hour blocks – for example, from 6.30 a.m. to 11.30 p.m. Then simply record in each half-hour block how you spend your time on different activities over a seven-day period. The choice of what kinds of activity to record is up to you, but you will find it useful to choose between, say, six and 12 different activities to cover your time both at work and outside.

Making explicit the time devoted to different activities often yields surprises and acts as a stimulus for making changes to focus on more important, satisfying or enjoyable activities. You may be surprised to discover, for instance, how much time you spend watching TV or in meetings or doing household chores, and perhaps how little time you spend doing things for yourself that you really enjoy. With this awareness, you might then make some decisions about how you want to spend your time differently.

Table 8.1 An example of a time log

	Day 1	Day 2	Day 3	Day 4	Day 5	Day 6	Day 7
6.30							
7.00							
7.30							
8.00							
8.30							
9.00							
9.30							
10.00							
10.30							
11.00							
11.30							
12.00							
12.30							
1.00							
1.30							
2.00							
2.30							
3.00							
3.30							
4.00							
4.30							
5.00							
5.30							
6.00							
6.30							
7.00							
7.30							
8.00							
8.30							
9.00							
9.30							
10.00							
10.30							
11.00							
11.30							

Exercise 8.2 Your time log

Copy out the log in Table 8.1 on the previous page to keep a simple record of how you spend your time over seven typical days. This should cover both work activities and non-work activities, and should also include both weekdays and weekend.

Record approximately how much time you spend each day on different kinds of activity. The choice of what kinds of activity to record is entirely up to you – choose categories that make sense to you in your job and outside work. It is probably useful to have, say, between six and 12 areas of activity. You can ignore time spent sleeping, unless this is an area that is problematic for you.

When you have completed your log, add the total time you spend on each activity. Then consider these questions:

- Which areas of activity take up a lot of time but are not that important to you?
- Which areas of activity are important to you but are not given enough time?
- What are the main imbalances in how you split your time between work and non-work activities?
- What changes will you make to how you spend your time?

Delegation

A very good illustration of an activity that is important but often not urgent is delegating tasks to other people. Stephen Covey writes that 'effectively delegating to others is perhaps the single most powerful high-leverage activity there is'. Investing the time to effectively delegate a task to someone else frees you to spend your time on more important tasks.

The ability to delegate effectively is one of the most important skills in managing people. However, you might also delegate tasks to other family members, people in your social circle, or fellow volunteers in a charity or committee.

People who find it difficult to delegate frequently give excuses such as the following:

- I don't have time to delegate.
- I don't have anyone to delegate to.

- It's too risky to delegate this.
- Other people are already overloaded.

There are occasions when each of these excuses is absolutely valid and constitutes a reason rather than an excuse for not delegating. But I suspect not nearly as often as people think.

Other reasons for not delegating, which may be true but are less likely to be admitted to, include:

- I don't trust other people.
- I can do it better or quicker myself.
- I like doing this task.
- I enjoy helping people.

What reasons or excuses do you yourself use for not delegating?

In the next chapter on achieving things through other people we offer some guidelines on how to delegate effectively. The ability to do this is a vital skill in managing your time. Taking time to delegate a task effectively can be a great investment of time which pays off not only in the time you subsequently save but also because it can build the capability and confidence of the person to whom the task is delegated. Moreover, if you can delegate effectively you are freed up to work on more important or strategic tasks – or to create a healthier work–life balance for yourself. When effective delegation becomes the norm within a team, it can help to create a culture of empowerment.

Handling emails

The 7 Habits of Highly Effective People was first published in 1989 and in it Covey doesn't mention emails, which cause many people big difficulties in managing their time today. I don't think that society has come to terms with the implications for work–life balance of email, mobile phones, the internet and social networking media. A generation or two ago, if you left the office at the end of the day you were finished with work unless you packed some things in your briefcase. Nowadays, you are free to work and perhaps to be contacted 24 hours a day, seven days a week.

We've moved now into the territory of tips to manage your time more effectively rather than the philosophical territory covered above. In this section I'd like to offer some tips to handle emails as part of time management.

I sometimes run a lunchtime workshop called Clear Your Inbox. The idea behind the workshop comes from a book by Declan Treacy called *Clear Your Desk*. He argues that you should only have on your desk the papers that relate to the task you are currently doing. When you are ready to move on to the next task, put those papers in your filing system and bring out the papers for the new task. Otherwise, if you have papers relating to a number of tasks on top of your desk, you will from time to time pick up unrelated paperwork and spend some time looking at it but not make any decisions. In this way you will waste several minutes and divert your attention from what you meant to work on. Over the course of a day – or a year – you'll waste lots of time and continually lose focus. So, Treacy recommends, clear your desk!

I've adapted Treacy's idea of clearing your desk to help me manage my emails. Let me begin by suggesting that there are only four things you can do with an email:

1 Delete it.
2 Reply to it.
3 Forward it.
4 File it – and put on your 'to do' list.

Let's look at these four possibilities in turn.

1 Many emails – spam is the obvious but not the only example – don't require you to do anything. Delete them straight away.
2 Some emails require a quick reply which may take you seconds or perhaps a few minutes. Reply to them now. File if necessary.
3 Other emails require a response from someone else. Forward the email to the right person and delegate the task. File if necessary.
4 Some emails create work for you. One of the features of emails is that two lines of text might generate months of work. You can't deal with such an email now. Put it on your 'to do' list – mine is paper based but yours might be electronic or even simply in

your head. You're going to have to refer to this email again, so file it where you can find it.

If you adopt this practice, then you can clear your inbox. You'll find this is far more effective than having an inbox full of dozens or even hundreds of emails that you have looked at but not dealt with – alongside all the new emails that have arrived since you last looked. And you won't waste time glancing guiltily at all those emails that do need attention, but not now.

To make this approach work, you need two things: a 'to do' list that works for you and an email filing system that works for you. I suggest that an important but not urgent task is to set up your email filing system, which is a useful investment of time that will save far, far more time in the long run.

I also find that it's useful to clear my Sent box several times a day. I reckon that 90 per cent of the emails I send don't need filing and so can be deleted, and that I know immediately where to file the others if I've just been working on them. I can then easily retrieve these emails later if necessary.

Note that clearing your inbox in this way doesn't stop the emails arriving in the first place. That's a different problem!

Another tip for managing the time you spend on emails is to deal with them at specific times rather than continually through the day. Depending on the nature of your role, this might be one or more times a day, and certain times of the day will suit you better than others. And I do suggest that you silence the noise and disable the pop-up that tells you a new email has arrived, seducing you from the task that you wanted to focus on.

Eat that frog

Here is another simple idea that may help you manage your time better. Identify – possibly from your time log – the things that waste your time. Here are some common timewasters, some of which we've mentioned above:

- Frequent interruptions – telephone or other
- Shuffling paperwork around

- A cluttered home or office
- Meetings that are too long or not really necessary
- Office or household procedures not properly set up
- Trying to do to much – unable to say no
- Inability to delegate effectively or to ask for help
- Procrastination.

Which of these ways of wasting time afflict you personally? What can you do to address this?

Brian Tracy's book *Eat That Frog* offers a way of dealing with the last of these timewasters, procrastination or putting things off till another time. Most of us are unlikely to put off the jobs that are interesting and enjoyable. Rather, it is the difficult or unpleasant tasks that we are more likely to postpone. A difficult conversation, setting up a filing system or making an appointment to see the dentist might be examples of unpleasant tasks. Other tasks might be difficult because they are large and important. Tracy calls these tasks that we need to do 'frogs'. He recommends:

- The key to reaching high levels of performance and productivity is to develop the habit of tackling your major task first thing each morning.
- Eat your frog before you do anything else and without taking too much time to think about it.

A colleague who spent some time in Washington working with political advisers gave me a good example of eating a frog. Candidates for political office in the USA need to raise significant amounts of money to fund their campaigns. One of the things they most dislike doing is making the phone call to a potential donor to ask for financial support. It's a frog! And their advisers will push them to make that call early in the day so that it's over and done with, freeing them to focus their attention without being distracted by the negative emotions felt when thinking about unpleasant jobs still to be tackled.

Tracy goes on to advise what to do if you have two unpleasant or difficult tasks:

- If you have to eat two frogs, eat the uglier one first. In other words, start with the biggest, hardest and most important task.

Exercise 8.3 Eat that frog

- What are the difficult or unpleasant tasks that you have been putting off?
- What is the biggest and ugliest of these frogs?
- When are you going to eat that frog?

9

Achieving things
through other people

Introduction

In this chapter we focus on situations where you want to achieve things through the efforts of other people. It may be that you are a line manager or supervisor with responsibility for managing a number of people within an organization. Or perhaps you chair the local branch of a charity, run a local sports team or are a teacher in charge of a project with a group of students. Although we won't focus on this in the chapter, if you are a parent you might reflect on how you could use some of the ideas with your children.

We begin with the idea that, in seeking to achieve things through others, you need to balance concern for completion of the task and looking after the people who are doing it. We then extend this to include the importance of managing the team collectively as well as the task and the individual people. We consider a definition of when a group is in fact a team, and look at a model of how teams develop. We end the chapter by comparing management with leadership, suggesting that to be successful you need a blend of both management and leadership.

Concern for task and concern for people

Robert Blake and Jane Mouton developed a simple framework which they called the managerial grid. As illustrated in Figure 9.1, this proposes that when you are looking to achieve things through other people then you have to balance concern for the task and concern for the people involved.

If you concentrate exclusively on making sure that the task is completed – maybe in a somewhat cold or unfeeling way – then you may not get the full commitment of the people who might, therefore, not contribute as much as they are capable of. On the other hand, if you focus on trying to ensure that everyone is happy, you may fail to accomplish what you set out to do.

In fact, there isn't necessarily a trade-off between addressing the needs of the task and the needs of the people. A really successful leader understands that the task is achieved through the efforts of the people involved, and will spend time addressing both sets of needs.

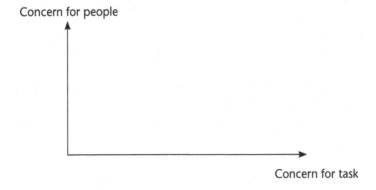

Figure 9.1 Concern for task and concern for people

The managerial grid can be related to the Theory X and Theory Y view of motivation developed by Douglas McGregor. If you take a Theory X view of people, you assume that people are inherently lazy, dislike work and seek to avoid responsibility. With this view of the world, you are unlikely to trust people. If incentives and punishments are available to you, you are likely to use a mix of carrot and stick to ensure compliance with your instructions or orders. An authoritarian manager who sees his or her role as to command, control and direct others probably holds a Theory X view of people.

In contrast, if you have a Theory Y view of people you believe that people enjoy work and are talented, creative and able to motivate themselves. You reckon that people want to do a good job, and that this in itself can be motivating. Hence you are likely to communicate openly, share decision-making and generate a climate of trust. Holding a Theory Y belief in people is a great asset if you want to meet the needs of both the task and the people at the same time.

Exercise 9.1 Concern for task and for people

Think of some situations where you are seeking to achieve an outcome that is dependent on the commitment and abilities of other people.

- On a scale of 1 (not at all) to 10 (to a great extent), how much thought and time do you give to ensuring that the task is completed successfully?
- On a scale of 1 (not at all) to 10 (to a great extent), how much care and attention do you give to ensuring that the people are feeling involved and satisfied?
- To what extent do you hold a Theory X or a Theory Y view of people in general and of the people that you yourself lead?
- What might you do differently to meet the needs of both task and people simultaneously?

Task, team and individual

Although John Adair developed what he terms his action-centred model of leadership independently of Blake and Mouton's managerial grid, I think of his framework as adding an extra dimension to their notion of concern for task and for people. Adair suggests that an effective leader needs to allocate time to

- ensure the **task** is completed;
- keep the group or **team** working together;
- meet the **individual** needs of each team member.

Let's now explore some of the things you might do when you are leading a group of people to address the needs of the task, the individuals and the team.

Completing the task

To ensure that tasks are completed effectively and efficiently, Adair says that you have to:

- specify and agree objectives;
- allocate resources;
- review progress;
- evaluate performance.

I think the first point is fundamental. It is vital that people are clear about what you're asking them to achieve. This seems obvious, but in many situations people are not at all clear what they are expected to deliver.

A commonly used mnemonic is that objectives need to be SMART. There are various versions of what these five letters mean, but typically SMART objectives are:

- Specific
- Measurable
- Achievable
- Relevant
- Time bounded.

While I think that it is often useful to have objectives which are SMART, and that this is a helpful checklist when setting objectives, I also believe that there are times when objectives are necessarily and usefully somewhat fuzzy and where the attempt to make them SMART is unduly constraining. As an illustration, let's imagine that you have just bought a house with a large and somewhat neglected garden. As a keen gardener, you have many ideas about how you'd like to develop the garden. On moving into the house you may well know some of the things you want to create – borders with shrubs and flowers, a vegetable patch, some fruit trees, and so on – but at this point you're not ready to be specific. You want to live in the house for a 12-month cycle to find out more about the plants that are already there. At a later date it will be useful to be explicit about what exactly you want to do in each area of the garden, and to set yourself goals and deadlines as the seasons unfold. But at the time of moving in, while you have some definite ideas to work on, you're not ready to specify your objectives in SMART terms.

Having set the objectives or agreed them with the people involved, it is important also to monitor progress. How closely you check on the work being done by others depends on a number of factors. You may well have your own style – some people are happy to trust folk to get on with things while others must know in detail how things are progressing. Some of the people helping you may be experienced and confident, and can largely be left to get on with things. However, there may be others who are lacking in skill or commitment and so need much closer monitoring. Moreover, the importance of the task is relevant too – you may well monitor more closely a task that is crucial to the overall success of your project and be more relaxed about one which is less significant.

I would make one brief comment about allocating resources. As with setting objectives, the necessity of this seems both obvious and fundamental. However, I have observed on numerous occasions people being asked to do a task without being given sufficient resources – people, budgets, equipment – to do the job properly.

Meeting the needs of individuals

If you are leading a group of people, Adair suggests that you have to:

- treat each member as an individual;
- acknowledge different opinions, work styles and motivation;
- encourage each individual to contribute fully;
- keep individuals informed;
- provide development opportunities according to individual needs.

An example of someone who was great at treating people as individuals was the England cricket captain Mike Brearley. He was by no means the most talented batsman in the side, but he was able to read people well and tailor his approach to get the most from each of the players. Interestingly, he went on to become a psychotherapist.

One of the most important ways in which you develop effective working relationships with people is through the conversations you have with them. In Chapter 5 on conversations we explored the four key skills of conversation – listening, playing back, questioning and voicing.

I find the idea of the coaching dance a very useful framework for thinking about how the nature of the conversation needs to shift when you are trying to achieve results through other people. It was devised by David Hemery, an Olympic gold medallist in the 400 metres hurdles in 1968, who has helped many people learn how to coach. He describes how you can move from 'tell' to 'ask', and back again.

As an illustration, you might tell someone explicitly what you require ('I must have the report by 3.00 on Friday') and then ask them how they can achieve it ('What do you need to do to finish this by Friday?'). Hemery calls it a dance because when you do this well you are moving skilfully and gracefully between telling and asking. In the example, if the report really has to be with you by 3.00 on Friday then it's unhelpful to ask 'When can you finish the report by?' in the hope that you'll be given the answer you require. Be clear what's given and what's up for discussion.

Delegation

We saw in the previous chapter that the ability to delegate tasks to other people is an important aspect of managing your time well. Moreover, delegating effectively is a key way in which you balance concern for task and concern for people.

Here are some guidelines on how to delegate a task successfully:

- Choose an appropriate person to delegate the task to.
- Explain clearly – so that the person understands – the outcome you are looking for.
- Be as precise as you feel it necessary to be about quality standards, constraints and deadlines.

- Don't tell the person how to do the task – let him use his initiative and creativity.
- Check that the person is committed to completing the task.
- Monitor progress appropriately – delegation isn't abdication – and be available to offer support if necessary.
- Review the task when it's completed and, if appropriate, help the person to distil what he has learnt.
- Say thank you.

I like the quote from the US Second World War general, George Patton, who said, 'Never tell people how to do things. Tell them what you want them to achieve and they'll surprise you with their ingenuity.'

You may also find the following checklist useful when you are asking someone to do something for you:

1 Is the person **clear** about what you're asking him or her to do?
2 Is he or she **capable** – perhaps with some training – of doing it?
3 Is he or she **confident** about taking it on?
4 Is he or she **committed** to doing the task?

You have to be able to tick all four points in order to feel confident delegating the job to that person. Moreover, you need to offer different interventions depending on where the gap is.

First of all, the person to whom the task is being delegated needs to be clear what you are asking her to do. Note that it's not enough that you are clear – what matters here is that the other person also is clear.

Second, if the person isn't capable of doing the task, then it's foolish to delegate it to her – unless you're going to help her develop her capability at the same time.

Third, the person may be clear and capable but lack confidence. In this case, you might delegate the task but need to offer appropriate support. Someone who successfully achieves the task in this situation may very well develop considerably.

Finally, if the problem lies in the person not feeling committed to the task, then the intervention you require is very different from in the other instances. I think that commitment and motivation ultimately come from within, so you'll need to consider what – if anything – will motivate this individual to take on responsibly this particular task.

Exercise 9.2 Delegating tasks

Think of a situation where you asked someone to do something for you and he or she didn't deliver satisfactorily. With hindsight, to what extent do you think that person was lacking in the following?

• clarity
• capability
• confidence
• commitment.

Keeping the team working together

To lead a team well, Adair suggests that you have to:

• ensure key roles are filled by appropriate people;
• build trust and inspire teamwork;
• deal with conflict;
• expand team capabilities;
• facilitate and support team decisions.

If you are a line manager, one of the most important ways in which you invest your time is interviewing to recruit a new member of the team. Recruiting someone who isn't suitable is a mistake that you may have to live with for a very long time. On the other hand, recruiting a talented and motivated person who is going to get on well with the rest of your team is one of the delights of the role.

Managing the dynamics within the team – handling conflict, dealing with rivalries, encouraging the more reticent to contribute, putting people with complementary styles together, and so on – is also part of your role as a leader. You may, as many people do, choose to ignore tensions, disagreements and rivalries within the team. But the performance of the team and the morale of the individuals within it will be influenced by the team dynamics, and you ignore it to your cost.

From time to time, conflict – which we defined in Chapter 7 as any form of disagreement, no matter how large or small – can emerge in the team. In a well-managed team conflict is acknowledged and worked through to find a way forward. In less healthy teams conflict gets ignored, which means that it persists and undermines morale and performance.

When you are leading a group of people you may not only wish to ensure that the team is working well together to achieve their current set of objectives but you may also be seeking to build its overall effectiveness and capability. Just as individuals learn from reflecting on their experiences, so too a team collectively can learn from their performance. One of the ways in which they can do this is to review together how things went – both the positives and the negatives – and learn from their shared experiences. When you facilitate this kind of review effectively, you can help the team to learn, address and resolve conflict, and build morale and team spirit.

What is a team?

This raises the question of what makes a group of people a team. In their book *The Wisdom of Teams* Jon Katzenbach and Douglas Smith offer a very useful definition of a team:

> A team is a small number of people with complementary skills committed to a common purpose, performance goals and ways of working together for which they hold themselves mutually accountable.

I think it is worth studying the various phrases which make up the definition, all of which are carefully chosen. For me, the key phrase is 'mutually accountable'.

I find that the definition is liberating. There are many groups who work together reporting to the same manager but who are not and need not be a team. I remember facilitating a team-building away-day for a group of managers in a large industrial company. Each of them reported to the same director, but they had very different responsibilities – finance, human resources, purchasing, legal, and so on. They had certain needs to communicate with one another as senior managers in the organization and they shared a boss, but they did not need to struggle to be a team – or indeed go on an away-day together. Each of the managers, however, was the leader of a team – that is, a group of people mutually accountable for delivering results – within his or her own function.

If you lead a group of people, you might like to consider to what extent they are genuinely a team according to Katzenbach and Smith's definition.

Stages of team development

There are a variety of models of how teams develop. The most widely quoted is Bruce Tuckman's 'Forming, Storming, Norming, Performing' model. However, I think its popularity owes more to the memorability of the mnemonic rather than its accuracy as a model. For example, while some groups do go through a Storming stage as people vie for position, I don't think it's inevitable that this has to occur.

Tuckman's original 1965 formulation was based on a survey of 50 articles on group development, and three-quarters of these studies were based on therapy groups or encounter groups. It is not obvious that the stages of development of these groups will necessarily be the same as those of, for instance, a project group with a designated leader or a group of singers with a conductor.

In *Coaching for Performance* John Whitmore describes a model of team development that makes more sense to me. This suggests that teams go through three stages:

- inclusion
- assertion
- co-operation.

In the inclusion stage, people are gauging to what extent they are included in the group. They may be feeling insecure, and possibly asking themselves if they want to be in this group. Some people will deal with their anxiety about acceptance or rejection by being quiet or tentative, while others may compensate by being vocal or forceful.

In the assertion stage, people who feel included begin to assert themselves in order to stake a claim for their territory within the group and their place in the pecking order. There may be power struggles and lots of competition within the group. This can make the group productive. Many groups do not advance beyond this stage.

In the co-operation stage, people who feel established begin to support each other and to trust each other. There is a lot of commitment to the team, patience and understanding of each other, and humour and enthusiasm. There is also a willingness to challenge ideas, debate issues constructively and resolve conflict. The team is aligned well towards the achievement of its goals.

Note that it is entirely possible that a team will slip backwards at times to earlier stages of development. I like the way that the three stages are linked to the feelings and behaviours of individual members, which strikes me as a realistic basis for a model of group development.

If someone new joins a team – even one that is co-operative – that individual will still need to go through the inclusion and assertion stages, and this might affect how others behave. And a long-standing member of the team might revert back to the inclusion stage when a new leader or colleague joins the team.

Exercise 9.3 Where is your team?

Here is an exercise to explore where the individuals that make up a team that you lead – or are a member of – sit on the spectrum from inclusion through assertion to co-operation.

Make a list of the individuals in the team. Then take your notebook or a sheet of paper and draw three concentric circles, as shown in Figure 9.2.

Write the name of each member and yourself at appropriate points on the chart to reflect where you see each one on the spectrum and also their relative closeness to one another.

Take some time to reflect on why you have placed people where you did.

What actions or conversations need to happen to support individuals and to move the team forward?

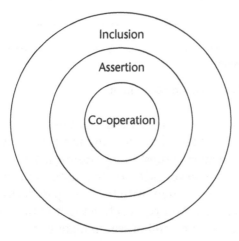

Figure 9.2 Inclusion, assertion and co-operation

A decision-making continuum

Warren Schmidt and Robert Tannenbaum described the continuum of leadership styles shown in Figure 9.3, in which at one end of the spectrum the team leader makes the decision alone and at the other the team is free to decide. It can be helpful to realize that these options are available to you. Which option you choose depends on the situation you are in and on the capability of the team.

1 You take the decision and announce it.
2 You decide and then sell your decision to the team.
3 You present the decision with background ideas and invite questions.
4 You suggest a provisional decision and invite discussion about it.
5 You present the problem or situation, get suggestions, and then decide.
6 You explain the situation or problem, define the parameters, and ask the team to decide on the solution.
7 You allow the team to identify a problem, develop options, and decide on the solution.

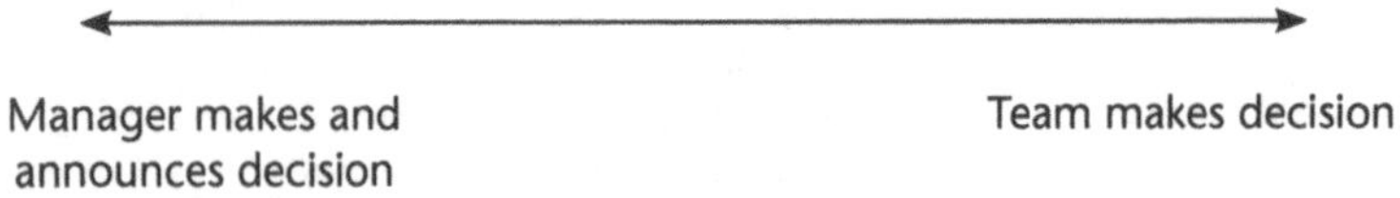

Manager makes and   Team makes decision
announces decision

Figure 9.3 Decision-making continuum

As an illustration of the continuum, imagine that you are the coach of a local football team. Choosing the 11 players who will take the field, and making substitutions during a match, are likely to be decisions that you yourself take. In setting tactics for a game, you might well discuss options with the team, particularly its more experienced members. And you could leave it entirely up to the team where to go for their end-of-season night out.

The continuum can be a useful guide when you are chairing a meeting. There may be some items where you are simply announcing a decision and others where you are genuinely consulting the group. It saves the time and energy of all concerned if you are clear about this. As we discussed in the coaching dance, it is useful to be clear when you are telling and when you are asking. There may also be items where you are looking for the group to make a collective decision that everyone is committed to.

Exercise 9.4 What is your decision-making style?

Think about a team that you lead or a meeting that you chair regularly.

- Where do you generally operate on the decision-making continuum?
- Which parts of the continuum do you usually avoid?
- What changes will you make to your decision-making style?

Management and leadership

So far in this chapter I have deliberately used the words 'manager' and 'leader' without differentiating between them. John Kotter argues that it is in fact important to distinguish between management and leadership.

In Kotter's view, management is about coping with complexity. Good management brings order and consistency and promotes stability. Managers make plans and handle budgets; they create organization charts which they then staff; and they ensure that plans are carried out through controls, monitoring processes and problem-solving.

Leadership, on the other hand, is about coping with change, which becomes vital for survival in a volatile and highly competitive world. Leaders initiate change by developing a vision of the future and strategies to accomplish this vision; they communicate the vision skilfully; and they motivate and inspire people to buy into their vision.

Since leadership is about change and management is about dealing with the status quo, you may need to act as a leader far less often than as a manager. For most of the time you want to conduct your activities efficiently and effectively rather than change what you and your team are trying to achieve.

Kotter argues that while management and leadership have different purposes, both are essential. As an illustration, when President Kennedy said in the early 1960s that the United States would put a man on the moon by the end of the decade, that is an example of a leader painting an inspiring vision. To make the vision the reality it became when Neil Armstrong landed on the moon in 1969, a lot of management had to have taken place in the meantime.

The President of the United States has vast resources at his disposal. It's likely that you will have to do both the leadership and the management yourself. You may like to consider when you need to act as a leader and when you need simply to be a manager, and reflect on how much time you spend on the two activities.

10

Taking part in or chairing meetings

Introduction

There are many occasions when you have to attend a meeting in order to achieve a goal, resolve a disagreement, obtain information or move a project forward. You might have meetings that are more or less important with people such as your bank manager, your GP or medical consultant, a teacher of one of your children, a neighbour or a colleague involved in a sport or hobby that you pursue. In the first part of this chapter we shall look briefly at some ideas that may help you to prepare for a meeting, conduct the meeting well and follow up effectively after the meeting.

In the second half of the chapter we expand these ideas on what you can do before, during and after a meeting to a situation where you are chairing a meeting of a group of people. Perhaps you chair a local voluntary group or parent–teacher association, lead a choir or sports team, or manage a group of employees within an organization. In both work and non-work contexts, poorly managed meetings are very common, waste a lot of time, and lower people's morale and commitment.

We shall revisit some of the ideas from earlier chapters, particularly Chapter 5 on conversations. We also discuss two frameworks of David Kantor's that can help you to make sense of and manage what is happening within a meeting.

Preparing for a key meeting

One of Stephen Covey's seven habits of highly effective people that we looked at in Chapter 8 on time management is: begin with the end in mind. One thing you can very usefully do in preparing for a meeting is to be clear in your own mind what you want to achieve from it.

Gather together any information that you need for the meeting. For example, if you are going to see a local town councillor to ask her to intervene in a planning matter, collect and summarize the evidence that you want to share with her.

Think also about whether you wish the other person to prepare for the meeting too. For instance, if you are visiting a teacher to ask for additional support for one of your children, you might signal this in advance and provide him with relevant information about your child's situation.

When meeting a professional such as a lawyer, doctor or teacher, there is a risk that you might respond from your Adapted Child ego state if he or she begins to converse from a Parent ego state. Think about the frame of mind you want to be in, which may help you stay in an Adult ego state during the actual meeting. You might also wish to dress in a way which helps to set the tone you're looking for in the discussion.

Handling the meeting

Meetings are conversations. The four key skills that we looked at in Chapter 5 on conversations are invaluable in handling meetings well. It is vital that you can voice your thoughts assertively, giving the reasons for your views or explaining how you feel or asking for what you want. This enables you to put forward your thoughts clearly and confidently.

It may be important too to appreciate the other person's point of view. The other three conversational skills – listening to understand the other person's position, asking open questions to find out more about this, and playing back accurately so that he realizes you've understood his perspective – are very useful here.

The use of these conversational skills can enable you to behave with genuine assertiveness – stating your views clearly and allowing the other person to do so too. As mentioned above, staying in an Adult ego state without being intimidated into Adapted Child is tremendously helpful in meetings.

Another useful thing to do during or at the end of a meeting is to recap clearly what has been agreed, what decisions have been taken and who is responsible – and by when – for any follow-up actions.

After the meeting

It is sometimes useful to follow up a meeting with a written note summarizing what has been agreed. You may also need to monitor over the next few days or weeks whether any actions are indeed being carried out. Sometimes it's necessary too to have a further meeting to progress matters.

Exercise 10.1 Reflecting on a meeting

Think about a recent meeting you had with another individual which didn't go very well. With the benefit of hindsight:

- What might you have done better in advance of the meeting?
- How might you have behaved more effectively during the meeting?
- What could you have usefully done to follow up after the meeting?

Preparing to chair a meeting

In the next part of the chapter we shall consider the situation where you are chairing a meeting involving a number of people. All of the ideas just discussed are relevant here too, and we shall expand on some of the points.

As mentioned earlier, it is important in preparing for a meeting to be clear in your own mind what you want to achieve from it. For example, your purpose may be to share information with the group, to gather the views of others, or to make a decision. These are very different purposes, calling for different ways of managing the meeting when it takes place. Your purpose might also affect whom you invite to attend the meeting. Moreover, if the meeting is going to cover a number of topics, the purpose may well vary from topic to topic.

It is very useful to have an agenda for the meeting. This may simply be some thoughts in your head or a few points on your notepad, or it may be a formal document circulated in advance to those attending. The agenda should reflect your objectives in holding the meeting. I would offer two suggestions about an agenda. First, be realistic in how many items you put on the agenda – a common mistake is to have an agenda that is unrealistically long.

Second, put the important items near the top of the agenda – if the meeting overruns then you are more likely to have covered the important items before time runs out. If different people will be present for different agenda items, then this too might influence the running order within the agenda.

A mundane point is to set a start time for the meeting. People will work out very quickly whether your meetings start on time or whether it's fine to turn up ten minutes late because you invariably wait for them to arrive. This punishes those who turn up on time. While it's important to allow for exceptions, I think it's helpful to start your meetings regularly on time. In a work context, it's important to set a finish time too – and once again to try to stick to it. Another mundane point, which can sometimes be problematic, is to arrange a suitable venue and, if required, appropriate refreshments or equipment.

Think too about whether or not you wish people to prepare for the meeting. You may want them to read some papers or to give some thought to some key issues or to put together information to be presented at the meeting. Specify clearly what you want people to do before the meeting. You'll probably find that some do what you ask and some don't! A common failing is to send out the papers for a meeting at the last minute, when people don't have sufficient time to read – never mind digest – the information sent. You also need to master your own briefs too before the meeting – make sure you've done your own preparation and reading!

Another thing to consider in advance of a meeting is whether you wish to influence some of the participants so that they support the case you wish to make. Think about the individuals who will be attending, their priorities and any tensions between different parties. It is generally better to lobby people, to bargain and, if you can, to resolve differences before the meeting takes place than to have the meeting dissolve into argument and conflict. Note, however, that there may be occasions when the purpose of the meeting is actually to explore and attempt to resolve differences.

Chairing the meeting

In Chapter 9, on achieving things through other people, we looked at the idea of a coaching dance where you move between telling and asking. We also looked at a continuum of decision-making styles where you move from making the decision on your own to allowing the group to decide. When you are chairing a meeting it's very helpful to be clear whether you are announcing a decision you have already made, arguing for a position that you hope will prevail, genuinely consulting to listen to the views or ideas of others, or facilitating a conversation where you are relaxed about the specific decision that emerges from the discussion. Or you may simply be sharing information. Note, however, that meetings can be a very inefficient way of passing on information, which often is better disseminated in advance of a meeting by email, say, or in one-to-one conversations.

If you are in the chair at a meeting then you are balancing the needs of the task, the individuals present and the group as a whole. You have to attend to the dynamics of the group – which can be a major challenge in itself. It is very difficult to facilitate the discussion of an agenda item when at the same time you are arguing strongly for a particular position. One thing you might do in this situation is to ask one of the other participants to take the chair for this item.

A key aspect of managing the process is managing the time, balancing appropriate discussion of an agenda item with moving forward to cover the items further down the agenda. The agenda itself is a useful guide to help you to keep the meeting on track. As we saw in Chapter 5 on conversations, playing back what has been said can be a very effective way of managing a conversation. Summarizing a discussion or repeating explicitly a decision taken or an action point agreed is a useful way of signalling that it's time to finish one item and move on to the next. It's important too not to let the discussion drift back to items that have been satisfactorily covered earlier in the meeting – or to engage prematurely in discussion of items which appear later on in the agenda.

You are also trying to balance the contribution of different people, which may mean explicitly inviting someone who is inexperienced or lacking in confidence to contribute and limiting the air time taken by more verbose individuals. Handling people who speak lengthily or who drift off the point is often easier said than done! On some occasions it may be sufficient to play back accurately your understanding of someone's position, enabling the discussion to move on. But there may be times when you have to be very firm, possibly stating explicitly that you wish to hear from others or to move on to the next item on the agenda. This calls for sensitivity as there is a risk of damaging relationships.

In *Effective Leadership* Christopher Achua and Robert Lussier note the following five types of problem member that you may find in your meeting:

- **Silent** – which means that the group does not benefit from that person's input;
- **Talker** – who has something to say about everything, and may seek to dominate the conversation;
- **Wanderer** – who changes the subject and distracts the group from the agenda items;
- **Bored** – who is not interested or is preoccupied with something else, and who may feel superior;
- **Arguer** – who enjoys arguing for the sake of arguing, rather than constructively criticizing, and may be seeking attention.

They warn against embarrassing, intimidating or arguing with problematic group members in front of the group. Rather, you need to confront serious problem members individually outside of the meeting.

If you are leading a meeting with the team that you manage, this may be one of the main opportunities you have to establish and maintain your credibility with the team and to manage your relationships with the individuals within the team. Knowledge of the Myers-Briggs® personality type profiles of each team member can help you to manage the conversation. For example, you might wish to draw out the Introverts or rein in the Extraverts. Or you might seek to balance some people's needs for detail or planning with others' needs for flexibility. And so on.

You will be greatly helped when you are leading a meeting if those attending are skilled at being effective participants. If each of them takes care to prepare for the meeting, is able to listen with an open mind and to put forward his or her views clearly and assertively, and is willing to accept decisions and to take responsibility for carrying out any actions assigned to him or her, then your job as chair becomes infinitely easier. You might also like to consider how skilled you are when you are a participant in, rather than the chair of, a meeting.

As you can see, there are several aspects to think about when chairing a meeting. One thing which may help you is to ask someone else to take notes of the meeting, which relieves you of one task. It's important to choose someone whom you can trust to keep up with the discussion and to record decisions accurately. As we shall consider in the next section, the notes or minutes of a meeting can be important documents which affect what happens next. In more formal situations, it is vital to have a secretary to the meeting who is competent, trustworthy and with whom you can work effectively.

It is important at the end of the meeting or as the meeting unfolds to make clear what decisions have been taken, and who is responsible, by when, for any actions that have been agreed.

After the meeting

As just noted, the minutes of a meeting are sometimes very important. In many situations, a simple list of action points – who will do what and by when – is sufficient. Moreover, producing minutes which are a list of action points takes far less time than minutes which record the different views expressed in a discussion. My own preference when I have to write minutes or notes of a meeting is to do this as soon as possible after the meeting, ideally immediately afterwards. I find that leaving it for a few days means that it takes me far longer to make sense of my notes and to remember some of the details. Circulating a list of actions soon after a meeting also gives people more time to carry out the actions for which they are responsible. Depending on the situation, you may leave it to whoever took the notes to circulate these, or you may wish carefully to control what is issued.

Another aspect to consider after a meeting is follow-up conversations. You may need to pacify, reassure or encourage someone who has been upset by what took place. You may need to have a word with someone whose behaviour or contribution was unhelpful. Or you may need to offer practical support to someone to whom an important task has been assigned.

It may also be important to monitor progress on the actions that were agreed at the meeting. It can be very frustrating to learn at the next scheduled meeting that some people haven't carried out the tasks assigned to them. You may well know already the people who will responsibly carry out actions without further prompting and those who will require repeated reminders.

Exercise 10.2 Chairing meetings

Think about a meeting that you lead. If you are a line manager, this might be your regular meeting with your team. Or it might be a meeting in a non-work context which you chair.

Produce your own checklist of bullet points to remind yourself what you will do to:

- prepare before the meeting;
- handle task, team and individual aspects during the meeting;
- follow up effectively after the meeting.

You might like to use the checklist from time to time to reflect upon your latest experiences of chairing meetings, and possibly modify your checklist in the light of your learning.

Three languages

In the remainder of the chapter we shall consider two frameworks described originally by David Kantor that offer ways of making sense of how people speak and act in meetings. We begin with his notion that people use one of three different languages to express themselves – power, meaning and affect (or feeling). See Figure 10.1.

- Someone who is using the language of **power** is interested in what we are going to do.

- Someone who is using the language of **meaning** is interested in the ideas and values behind what is happening.
- Someone who is using the language of **affect** is concerned about the feelings of the people involved and the relationships between them.

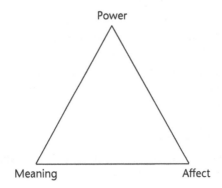

Figure 10.1 David Kantor's three languages

Here are three examples of contexts where I've encountered each of these languages. When I worked in the gas pipeline company Transco, the culture was dominated by the engineers whose activities were at the heart of the business. Transco engineers largely spoke what Kantor calls the language of power. They were most at home when they were active, making decisions and – sometimes literally – fighting fires. However, they could find it difficult to stand back and reflect using the language of meaning.

I now work at the University of Warwick where the culture is shaped by the academics who are the key players in the organization. Academics often talk in the language of meaning, and feel most comfortable debating ideas and producing alternative points of view. However, they can find it difficult to make a decision, particularly in a group.

From time to time I facilitate a supervision session for a group of people who teach counselling and psychotherapy. I've noticed that they naturally use the language of affect.

In *Dialogue and the Art of Thinking Together* Bill Isaacs writes of Kantor's three languages that:

These are in fact truly different languages: Communication across them carries the same difficulties that translation between any two languages carries. People speaking the language of feeling tend to be discounted by people who speak the language of action and power. Asking such people to reflect about the meaning of things can often evoke the reaction that you are being too 'intellectual'. And asking questions about how to take action may feel premature to those communicating via the language of feeling or meaning.

Recognizing the different languages that people tend to speak can be very useful when you are chairing a meeting. For example, if the purpose of the meeting or an agenda item is to make a decision, some people will be comfortable doing this while others may need you to focus their attention explicitly on the need for a decision.

Exercise 10.3 What language do you speak?

Copy out Figure 10.1 and place a cross somewhere in the triangle to represent the language that you yourself generally use. For example, if you use a combination of power and meaning with little or no affect, you might place the cross somewhere on the left-hand edge.

When you are in a situation where you are seeking to influence or negotiate with another person, consider which language that person is speaking. You may find it helps to put forward your views in the language which he or she uses rather than your own.

The four-player system

David Kantor describes a second framework, which he calls the four-player system, to explain different stances that people may take in a meeting (Figure 10.2 overleaf).

- When someone **moves**, he or she is proposing something or initiating an action.
- When someone **follows**, he or she is supporting a move.
- When someone **opposes**, he or she is challenging what is being said or proposed.

- When someone **bystands**, he or she is offering a perspective on what is happening in the conversation. (Note that the term 'bystanding' does not mean being uninvolved or silent.)

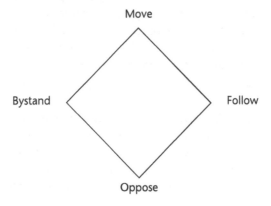

Figure 10.2 David Kantor's four-player system

To illustrate the four roles in the model, let's imagine that we are in a group discussing how we'll spend the evening. If I say, 'Let's go to the cinema', then I'm making a move. And if you reply, 'There's a really good film on at the Odeon', then you are following, seeking to build on my suggestion. However, if you say, 'Oh no, we went to the cinema last night', then you are opposing my idea. And if someone else says, 'That's the sixth idea we've looked at and we still haven't decided what to do tonight', he or she is making a bystanding comment.

David Kantor argues that a healthy conversation requires all of these roles to be played. Moreover, everyone in the conversation is free to occupy any of the four positions. A team in which it isn't acceptable to oppose the views of the leader or to make a bystanding comment when the group is stuck is likely to be both unhealthy and less than fully productive.

Being aware of the value of all four types of contribution – and using this to draw out different perspectives – can be very helpful when you are chairing or simply taking part in a meeting of a group of people.

Exercise 10.4 Which positions are missing?

Think about meetings at work or outside where you collaborate with a particular group of people. Reflect on the conversations that typically take place when that group comes together.

- Which of the move, follow, oppose and bystand positions dominate the conversation?
- Which positions are largely missing from the discussion?
- Which of the stances do you yourself typically take in these meetings?
- To enhance the effectiveness of these meetings, what might you do differently?
- What might others do differently?

11

Coping with
and introducing change

Introduction

Change is a common aspect of life today. Behind this simple statement lie countless individual stories of worry and fear, confusion
and anger, excitement and possibility, and growth and development. In the first half of the chapter we shall explore a number of
models that help to make sense of change, inviting you to reflect
upon how you and other people cope with change. In the second
half we consider a number of ideas that may help you if you are
the person introducing a change that may affect others. We also
look at the situation of a middle manager who may at one and the
same time be implementing someone else's change ideas, seeking
to introduce change, and coping with the possibility that she
herself is a potential casualty of change.

The change curve

Elisabeth Kübler-Ross was a Swiss psychiatrist who worked with
terminally ill cancer patients. In her book *On Death and Dying* she
introduced the notion of five stages of grief, as shown in Figure
11.1.

- Denial – This isn't happening to me.
- Anger – Who's to blame for this? Why me?
- Bargaining – If I can live till my daughter's wedding . . .
- Depression – I am too sad to do anything.
- Acceptance – I'm at peace with what is coming.

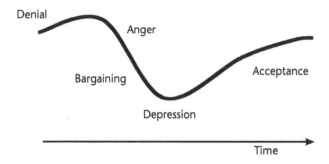

Figure 11.1 The Kübler-Ross grief curve

Note that there is no single or simple path through these five stages. The different stages can be experienced many times, they may come in a different order, and sometimes several of the stages are experienced at the same time.

Her theory, which applies to the phases of grief a dying person goes through, has often been misunderstood and applied to family or friends grieving the death of another person. Kübler-Ross's original model has been modified many times, and numerous versions of the change curve have been produced.

In an article called 'Beyond the Peter Principle – managing successful transitions', Chris Parker and Ralph Lewis describe a transition curve which includes seven stages experienced by someone who has been promoted. This can serve as a model to help make sense of other experiences of change or loss (see Figure 11.2 overleaf). Note that some changes are positive and some are negative. Moreover, some changes are planned and some are unplanned. For example, getting married is usually a planned and positive experience, whereas the sudden death of a relative or friend is an unplanned and negative experience.

Exercise 11.1 Examples of change

Make a list of the significant changes that have affected you in your life.

- Which of these changes were generally positive and which were generally negative?

- Which changes were planned and which were unplanned?
- Which changes are difficult to categorize in these ways?

You may find that some changes feel more positive or negative with hindsight than they did at the time.

Parker and Lewis's seven stages are:

1 Immobilization or shock – a sense of being overwhelmed
2 Denial of change – minimizing or trivializing the change
3 Incompetence and depression – with flat performance, frustration, difficulty in coping
4 Accepting reality – letting go of the past and accepting the situation
5 Testing – trying new approaches and behaviours
6 Search for meaning, internalization – a reflective period with an attempt to understand all that has happened
7 Integration – incorporating new meanings into new and enhanced behaviours.

Parker and Lewis also note that not everyone will follow this general curve and that different people will experience unique progressions and regressions depending on their circumstances.

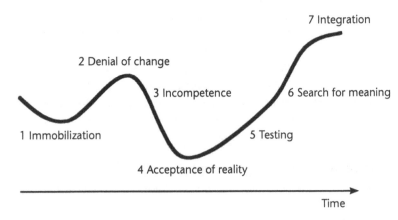

Figure 11.2 Parker and Lewis's transition curve

There are other versions of the change curve that have similarities with Kübler-Ross's original version and the Parker and Lewis model. People often find it reassuring to know that going through a range of thoughts and emotions when coping with change – even a planned or desired change – is a common experience. It also helps to know that the process takes time, and that slipping back along the curve is normal too.

Exercise 11.2 Coming to terms with change

Choose one of the significant changes in your life that you listed in Exercise 11.1. Take a sheet of paper and draw a line to represent the passage of time as you went through the change curve in that situation. Make some notes to capture your thoughts and feelings and how these shifted over time.

Looking back on this experience, what lessons do you draw that will help you to plan for and deal with future changes?

Change and transition

In his book *Managing Transitions: Making the most of change* William Bridges draws a distinction between change and transition. He suggests that change is a shift in the externals of a situation – moving to a new home, starting college or being made redundant, for instance. Transition, on the other hand, is psychological. It is the 'process that people go through as they internalize and come to terms with the details of the new situation that the change brings about'. He argues that it is vital to understand and take account of transition if you want to make sense of how you are responding to a change or if you want to lead others through change.

Transition is the mental and emotional transformation that people go through as they relinquish old arrangements and embrace new ones. Bridges writes that it is 'a gradual psychological process through which individuals and groups reorient themselves so they can function and find meaning in a changed situation'.

He argues that transition consists of three phases – the ending, the neutral zone and the beginning. Paradoxically, change starts with ending and finishes with beginning (Figure 11.3 overleaf).

1 In the **ending** phase, each individual involved is trying to understand what has ended and to face up to the nature of his or her loss. There is likely to be a fear of the unknown. It is important to appreciate that this will result in resistance. Some people may become stuck in this phase. Bridges advises that you will save yourself a lot of trouble if you remember that the 'first task of transition management is to convince people to leave home'.

2 In the **neutral** zone, the old way has ended but the new way is not established. This phase is characterized by uncertainty, disorientation, confusion and discomfort. However, Bridges suggests that in this phase there may be tremendous opportunity to create new ways of thinking and working.

3 In the **beginning** phase, certainty returns. People discover new energy, new purpose and new identity. The new way of working feels comfortable, and may even seem like the only possible way.

Note that these three stages may not be sharply delineated, and different people will move forward at different paces.

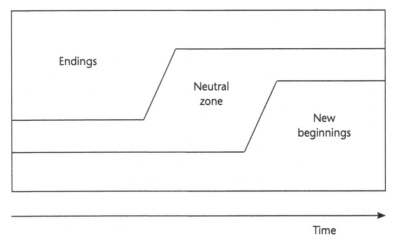

Figure 11.3 Bridges' transition curve

Individual responses to change

In his book *Diffusion of Innovations* Everett Rogers describes how different people respond to new ideas and technologies. As you read the descriptions which follow you might like to consider how you yourself adopted novel appliances such as personal computers or mobile phones. Rogers suggests that there are five types of people:

- Innovators – risk-takers who are the first to adopt new ideas
- Early adopters – willing to try out new ideas but in a more considered or careful way
- Early majority – thoughtful people who accept change more quickly than the average
- Late majority – sceptics who only change when everyone else has
- Laggards – traditional people who much prefer the 'old ways'.

In an analogous way people will respond at different rates to change. An individual's willingness to embrace change will also be affected by that person's past experiences of change, the extent to which he or she has voluntarily chosen the change, and his or her degree of involvement in introducing the change.

In his classic work on motivation, described in his 1954 book *Motivation and Personality* Abraham Maslow described a hierarchy of needs. Figure 11.4 overleaf shows a pyramid describing five levels of needs. (Incidentally, Maslow himself never represented his hierarchy as a pyramid, though many later writers have.) When physiological or safety needs at the lower levels are unmet, then the individual will focus all efforts on satisfying these needs. Only when the lower levels of need are satisfied will a person seek to satisfy the higher needs for belonging, esteem and self-actualization. The five levels in Maslow's hierarchy of needs are:

- Self-actualization – personal growth and fulfilment
- Esteem – achievement, status, respect of others, self-esteem
- Belonging – love, friendship, family
- Safety needs – health, security, employment, etc.

- Physiological needs – air, food and water, shelter, sleep, etc.

At times of significant change – for example, when someone's job and livelihood are at risk – people are likely to slip down the hierarchy of needs and be more concerned about putting food on the table and paying the mortgage than about their status or personal development. If they are confident that these needs will be met, then they turn to questions such as job satisfaction and career fulfilment.

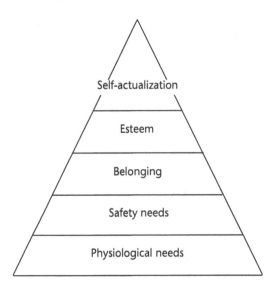

Figure 11.4 Maslow's hierarchy of needs

Exercise 11.3 How do you cope with change and transition?

Look back at Exercise 11.1, where you listed the significant changes that you have experienced. Reflect upon how you handled these various changes.

- On a scale of 1 (not at all) to 10 (very much), how readily do you respond to change?
- In Everett Rogers' terms, do you view yourself as an innovator, early adopter, early majority, late majority or laggard in how you embrace change?

Four options for change

Figure 11.5 shows a model which summarizes four generic options that are open to you if you find yourself in a situation that is unsatisfactory.

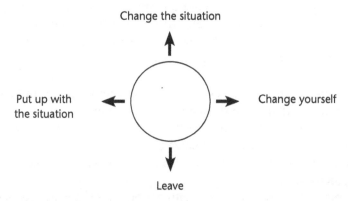

Figure 11.5 Four options for change

We'll illustrate the four options by assuming that you're in a situation where you're not happy with the house you're living in because it is too small.

1 One option is to leave – in this case, find another house with more space.
2 Another option is to change the situation – for example, you might build an extension.
3 A third option is to put up with the situation – stay in the house and continue to feel dissatisfied.
4 The final option is to change yourself – for example, rather than becoming frustrated and upset, tell yourself that this is a temporary situation and that when you can afford to you will find a larger house. Changing your attitude may reduce your feelings of dissatisfaction.

Note that the fourth option – changing yourself – is different from option 3 – putting up with the situation – since your thoughts and feelings are different in the two cases.

Leading and introducing change

In his book *Leading Change* John Kotter sets out the following eight-step model which offers a framework for someone wishing to lead a major organizational change. This may be a useful guide if, for instance, you are a head teacher looking to restructure teaching duties across your school, or an office manager seeking to introduce new technology and flexible working patterns, or a manager charged with merging two departments.

1 Establish a sense of urgency – identify external opportunities and threats that will motivate people to action.
2 Form a powerful guiding coalition – assemble a group with enough power to lead the change effort.
3 Create a vision – develop a vision and strategy to direct the change effort.
4 Communicate the vision – obtain the buy-in of as many people as possible through simple and frequent communication.
5 Empower others to act on the vision – remove obstacles to change, such as unhelpful systems or structures.
6 Plan for and create quick wins – set some manageable aims that are easy to achieve and visibly improve performance.
7 Consolidate improvements and produce more change – keep up the momentum of change with new projects.
8 Institutionalize new approaches – embed the changes in new behaviours and culture across the organization.

Kotter emphasizes that these phases in total take a considerable amount of time, and that skipping some of the steps never produces a satisfying result. He also points out that, as always, actions speak far louder than words. You might wish to adapt or simplify Kotter's framework if you yourself are in a position where you want to introduce a change that will affect other people.

Recall from Chapter 9 on achieving things through other people the need to balance concern for task and concern for people. If your Myers-Briggs Type Indicator® preference on the Thinking–Feeling dimension is T, you may well give priority to a logical analysis of the costs and benefits of the change, without necessarily considering the impact on the people involved and how you can get them on board. On the other hand, if your MBTI® preference is F, you may dilute or give up on the change that is necessary because you don't want to upset anyone. A useful combination is to work with a partner who has the opposite preference to you so that you adequately address both *what* you need to change and *how* you will bring people with you.

Change and the middle manager

The Kotter model is aimed at the leader who is initiating the change. If you are a middle manager or supervisor within an organization, there may be times when you yourself decide to introduce a change within your department or team, and the steps in Kotter's framework offer a framework to guide the various actions you need to carry out.

However, you may be in a position where the decision to change has been taken at some level above you in the hierarchy and your role is to implement the change within your area of the organization. You yourself may also be personally impacted by the change, with all the concerns that this raises. And you may have some scope to shape the detail of how the change initiative is translated into a new organizational structure within your own area. Hence, you may be at one and the same time:

- an implementer of someone else's change ideas;
- a shaper of change;
- a potential casualty of change.

Being in the middle during a change exercise is often uncomfortable. A common experience is that the people working for you think that you know what is happening and are keeping things from them, while you yourself are as much in the dark as they are. And there may also be times when you do have confidential information which you need to keep to yourself until a later date. It can be a very difficult place.

I worked in British Gas in the 1990s while the company went through a series of major organizational restructures as it adjusted to the consequences of being set up by the government in 1986 as a privatized monopoly. I recall one middle manager, a veteran of several restructures, saying to me: 'I can manage change – it's uncertainty I can't manage.' I think this frustration reflects the experience of many managers caught up in the middle of organizational restructures.

Creating a new structure

In this section we consider briefly the situation where you are faced with the challenge of restructuring your department. Let's suppose that the situation is such that you don't necessarily have to shed jobs, but rather you have to refocus the department to reflect shifts within the wider organization or in the external environment. Things are necessarily somewhat different when the reorganization has to yield significant savings of money and job losses.

The textbook guidance is to choose the structure you need and then to populate the roles in this structure through some combination of matching people to jobs and interviewing to fill posts. This makes logical sense – decide upon the roles that you need and then appoint people to these roles.

An alternative approach is to think first about the people in your department and then to build the structure around them. Early in my career I observed this taking place among the sales managers of the ICI division where I worked. At the time it struck me as favouritism. With the benefit of much more experience of organizational life, I now think there was a lot of merit in the approach. If people know that they will definitely have a place in the new structure, they are saved considerable worry and can get on with things. This reduction in personal and collective stress and uncertainty seems to me to have considerable benefits.

Moreover, it is often the case that a new organizational structure is simply different from, rather than better than, the old one. I recall a colleague from my time in the gas pipeline company, Transco – where there seemed to be a major organizational change every 18 months or so – saying wisely: 'With the right people, you'll make any structure work; with the wrong people it doesn't matter what structure you have.' I think many organizational changes take up vast amounts of time, emotion and money without yielding significant benefits – other than to the external consultants who were paid handsomely to redesign the organization! The example of the National Health Service comes to mind to illustrate the point.

Exercise 11.4 Introducing a change

Think of a change that you would like to introduce that will affect other people.

1 What is the change you want to make?
2 What are the likely benefits of this change?
3 What are the likely costs?
4 Whom do you expect to be in favour of the change? What can you do to enrol their active support?
5 Whom do you expect to resist the change? What are their concerns? What can you do to address each person's concerns?
6 What are the steps you will take, by when, to implement and to communicate the change?
7 When and how will you monitor progress?

Personal reflections on managing change

I'd like to end this chapter by offering a few suggestions based on my own experience as a member of staff caught up in the restructuring of several industrial corporations and on listening to coaching clients as they thought through how they were implementing or affected by organizational change.

- The most important question in change is: 'What does it mean for me?' When I am satisfied with the answer to this question, then I am able to think about what it means for others and for the organization.
- Treat people as adults. If my job is going to disappear, I want to know as early as possible so that I can take action to secure my future, pay my mortgage and look after my family.
- Communicate, communicate, communicate. And if you literally have nothing new to tell people, communicate this too.
- Act speedily. Once the decision to change has been made, implement the necessary actions quickly.

References

Achua, C. and Lussier, R. (2013) *Effective Leadership*. Mason, Ohio: South-Western, Cengage Learning.

Adair, J. (1979) *Action-Centred Leadership*. Farnborough: Gower.

Blake, R. and Mouton, J. (1964) *The Managerial Grid*. Houston: Gulf.

Bridges, W. (1991) *Managing Transitions: Making the most of change*. Reading, Mass.: Addison-Wesley.

Covey, S. (1989) *The 7 Habits of Highly Effective People*. London: Simon & Schuster.

Fisher, R. and Ury, W. (1997) *Getting to Yes: Negotiating an agreement without giving in*, second edition. London: Random House.

Goleman, D. (1996) *Emotional Intelligence*. London: Bloomsbury.

Harrison, R. (1995) *Consultant's Journey*. London: McGraw-Hill.

Hawkins, P. and Smith, N. (2006) *Coaching, Mentoring and Organizational Consultancy*. Maidenhead: Open University Press.

Isaacs, W. (1999) *Dialogue and the Art of Thinking Together*. New York: Currency Doubleday.

Karpman, S. (1968) 'Fairy tales and script drama analysis'. *Transactional Analysis Bulletin*, 7 (26), 39–43.

Katzenbach, J. and Smith, D. (1994) *The Wisdom of Teams*. New York: Harper.

Kotter, J. (1996) *Leading Change*. Boston: Harvard.

Kotter, J. (2001) 'What leaders really do'. *Harvard Business Review*, 79 (11), 85–98.

Kübler-Ross, E. (1969) *On Death and Dying*. New York: Macmillan.

McEwan, I. (1998) *The Innocent*. London: Jonathan Cape.

McGregor, D. (1960) *The Human Side of Enterprise*. New York: McGraw-Hill.

Maslow, A. (1954) *Motivation and Personality*. New York: Harper.

Myers, I. (1993) *Introduction to Type*. Oxford: Oxford Psychologists Press.

Myers, K. and Kirby, L. (2000) *Introduction to Type Dynamics and Development*. Oxford: Oxford Psychologists Press.

Newton, T. and Napper, R. (2010) 'Transactional Analysis and coaching', in E. Cox, T. Bachkirova and D. Clutterbuck (eds) *The Complete Handbook of Coaching*. London: Sage.

Parker, C. and Lewis, R. (1981) 'Beyond the Peter Principle – managing successful transitions'. *Journal of European Industrial Training*, 5 (6), 17–21.

Rogers, E. (1983) *Diffusion of Innovation*. New York: Free Press.

Schmidt, W. and Tannenbaum, R. (1960) *Management of Differences*. Los Angeles: University of California.

Smith, M. (1975) *When I Say No I Feel Guilty*. London: Bantam.

Stone, D., Patton, B. and Heen, S. (1999) *Difficult Conversations*. New York: Viking Penguin.

Thomas, K. and Kilmann, R. (1974) *Thomas–Kilmann Conflict Mode Instrument*. Mountain View, California: Xicom.

Tracy, B. (2001) *Eat That Frog*. San Francisco: Berrett-Koehler.

Treacy, D. (1998) *Clear Your Desk*. London: Arrow Business.

Tuckman, B. (1965) 'Developmental sequence in small groups'. *Psychological Bulletin*, 63 (6), 384–99.

Wheatley, M. (2002) *Turning to One Another*. San Francisco: Berrett-Koehler.

Whitmore, J. (2002) *Coaching for Performance*. London: Nicholas Brealey.

Index